MANAGING
HEART FAILURE IN
PRIMARY CARE

Managing Heart Failure in Primary Care

Edited by
H. J. Dargie, J. J. V. McMurray
& P. A. Poole-Wilson

Blackwell
Healthcare
Communications

This book is presented as a service to medicine by Bristol-Myers Squibb Pharmaceuticals Ltd. Sponsorship does not imply the sponsor's agreement or otherwise with the views expressed herein. Any product mentioned in this book should be used in accordance with the prescribing information prepared by the manufacturers.

© 1996 by
Blackwell Healthcare
Communications Ltd
Broadwalk Offices, 54 The Broadway
Ealing, London W5 5JN
An imprint of
Blackwell Science Ltd
Editorial Offices:
Osney Mead, Oxford OX2 0EL
25 John Street, London WC1N 2BL
23 Ainslie Place, Edinburgh EH3 6AJ
238 Main Street, Cambridge
  Massachusetts 02142, USA
54 University Street, Carlton
  Victoria 3053, Australia

Other Editorial Offices:
Arnette Blackwell SA
  224, Boulevard Saint Germain
  75007 Paris, France

Blackwell Wissenschafts-Verlag GmbH
  Kurfürstendamm 57
  10707 Berlin, Germany

  Zehetnergasse 6
  A-1140 Wien
  Austria

First published 1996

Set by Alden Multimedia Ltd
Printed and bound in Great Britain
at the Alden Press, Oxford and
Northampton

The Blackwell Healthcare
Communications logo is a trade mark of
Blackwell Science Ltd, registered at the
United Kingdom Trade Marks Registry.

DISTRIBUTORS
Marston Book Services Ltd
PO Box 269, Abingdon
Oxon OX14 4YN
(*Orders*: Tel: 01235 465500
          Fax: 01235 465555)

USA
Blackwell Science, Inc.
238 Main Street
Cambridge, MA 02142, USA
(*Orders*: Tel: 800 215-1000
                  617 876-7000
          Fax: 617 492-5263)

Canada
Copp Clark Professional
200 Adelaide Street, West, 3rd Floor
Toronto, Ontario M5H 17W
(*Orders*: Tel: 416 597-1616
                  800 815-9417
          Fax: 416 597-1617)

Australia
Blackwell Science Pty Ltd
54 University Street
Carlton, Victoria 3053
(*Orders*: Tel: 3 9347 0300
          Fax: 3 9347 5001)

A catalogue record for this title is available
from the British Library

ISBN 0-86542-966-9

Library of Congress
Cataloging in Publication Data

Dargie, Henry.
  Managing heart failure in primary care
  H.J. Dargie, J.J.V. McMurray,
  & P.A. Poole-Wilson.
      p.   cm.
  Includes bibliographical references
  and index.
  ISBN 0-86542-966-9
  1. Heart failure.
  I. McMurray, John.
  II. Poole-Wilson, Philip A.
  III. Title.
  [DNLM: 1. Heart Failure, Congestive.
  2. Primary Health Care.
  WG 370 D217m 1996]
  RC685.C53D37 1996
  616. 1′29—dc20
  DNLM/DLC
  for Library of Congress   96–27460CIP

Contents

Colour plates fall between pp. 84 and 85

List of Contributors

John Byrne *Department of Cardiology, Western Infirmary, Glasgow G11 6NT* [Chapter 13]

Henry J. Dargie *Clinical Research Initiative in Heart Failure, University of Glasgow, Glasgow G12 8QQ* [Chapters 1, 6, 7, 13]

Andrew P. Davie *Clinical Research Initiative in Heart Failure, University of Glasgow, Glasgow G12 8QQ* [Chapter 5]

Michael P. Love *Clinical Research Initiative in Heart Failure, University of Glasgow, Glasgow G12 8QQ* [Chapter 3]

Theresa A. McDonagh *Clinical Research Initiative in Heart Failure, University of Glasgow, Glasgow G12 8QQ* [Chapter 1]

John J.V. McMurray *Clinical Research Initiative in Heart Failure, University of Glasgow, Glasgow G12 8QQ* [Chapters 3, 5, 8, 10, 11]

Philip A. Poole-Wilson *Department of Cardiology, National Heart and Lung Institute, Imperial College, Dovehouse Street, London SW3 6LY* [Chapters 2, 4, 9, 12]

Stephen D. Robb *Department of Cardiology, Derby City General Hospital, Derby DE22 3NS* [Chapter 6]

Preface

Despite a continuing downward trend in the incidence of most cardiovascular diseases, heart failure is becoming a more common problem for doctors from several disciplines to deal with, as judged by the steady increase in hospital admissions, out-patient attendances and consultations in General Practice. Given that heart failure together with its asymptomatic precursor, left ventricular dysfunction, are as common as diabetes, and that both components are eminently susceptible to effective treatment in terms of reduction in morbidity and mortality, the scope for successful management in primary care is considerable.

Although this book is entitled *Managing Heart Failure in Primary Care*, it should be recognized that no artificial dividing line can reliably separate issues that are uniquely 'specialist' or 'generalist'. Thus the emphasis is on continuity with the identification of a basic core of knowledge that is a prerequisite for the optimum management of the complex condition currently known as 'heart failure'.

In this book experts from the UK address a spectrum of subjects relevant to management beginning with a modern view of the nature and scope of the condition as a prelude to the basis of its diagnosis, investigation, drug treatment and prevention.

Henry Dargie

What is Heart Failure?

SUMMARY POINTS

- Heart failure is a clinical syndrome, encompassing a wide range of pathophysiological states
- The main clinical manifestations of heart failure are breathlessness, fatigue and signs of fluid retention
- Different therapeutic strategies are required for acute heart failure, cardiogenic shock, high-output heart failure, right ventricular failure and chronic heart failure
- Chronic heart failure is the commonest manifestation of left ventricular dysfunction secondary to myocardial infarction

In pathophysiological terms, heart failure is 'a state in which an abnormality of cardiac function is responsible for failure of the heart to pump blood at a rate commensurate with the requirements of the metabolising tissues or, to do so, only from an elevated filling pressure'.[1] Although this terminology is useful for physiologists, the more pragmatic approach required by clinicians creates problems of definition.

The difficulty in clinically defining heart failure stems from the fact that it is not a diagnosis *per se*, but a clinical syndrome consisting of a constellation of symptoms and signs attributable, ultimately, to cardiac dysfunction. As such, it represents the ultimate expression of most serious forms of heart disease.[2]

> The difficulty in clinically defining heart failure stems from the fact that it is not a diagnosis *per se*, but a clinical syndrome

Thus, heart failure encompasses a wide spectrum of pathophysiological states ranging from those caused by rapid impairment of pump function, such as massive myocardial infarction and tachy- or bradyarrhythmias, to the progressive and gradual impairment of myocardial function observed in a patient whose heart is subjected to pressure or volume overload or who has a chronic intrinsic disorder of the heart muscle.

From a practical clinical point of view, heart failure is diagnosed when symptoms of breathlessness (either at rest or on exertion) or fatigue and signs of fluid retention (peripheral oedema, pulmonary crepitations or elevated jugular venous pressure) are found in a patient whom the clinician suspects of having heart disease.

Problems with definition

Historically, the concept of heart failure has been complicated by a plethora of descriptive terms related to involvement of the right or left ventricles, the acuteness or chronicity of the condition, and the presence of 'backward or forward failure'. As the following list illustrates, many are still in clinical use to describe the varying manifestations of heart failure that may require different therapeutic strategies:

Acute heart failure

This often refers to acute (cardiogenic) pulmonary oedema. Most commonly, it is a consequence of acute myocardial infarction (where there is extensive loss of ventricular muscle). However, acute heart failure may also occur following rupture of the interventricular septum and production of a ventricular septal defect. Alternatively, it may be due to acute valvular regurgitation, as is encountered in infective endocarditis.

Cardiogenic shock

Cardiogenic shock is a syndrome characterized by low systemic blood pressure, oliguria and poor peripheral perfusion. It usually occurs as a consequence of acute myocardial infarction and is associated with a high mortality.

High-output heart failure

High-output heart failure develops when the heart is unable to meet the excessive metabolic demands placed on it by conditions such as anaemia, thyrotoxicosis, beriberi, Gram-negative septicaemia, pregnancy, arteriovenous fistulae and Paget's disease of bone. It is in contrast to the low-output failure characteristic of most forms of chronic heart failure.

Right ventricular failure

This syndrome occurs in association with:
- chronic lung disease (when it is often referred to as cor pulmonale);
- pulmonary embolism or primary pulmonary hypertension;
- tricuspid or pulmonary valve disease;
- left-to-right shunts (atrial and ventricular septal defects);
- isolated right ventricular cardiomyopathy.

These variants of right ventricular dysfunction will not be considered in any further depth here. It is worth remembering that the most important and frequent cause of right ventricular failure is that which occurs secondary to left heart failure, also known as biventricular failure. For the present purposes, it is considered under the heading of chronic heart failure.

Other descriptive terms

Forward and backward failure

The distinction between forward and backward failure arose as a result of efforts to explain the symptoms and signs of heart failure. The backward theory contended that blood accumulated when a cardiac chamber failed to eject its contents fully, increasing the pressure in the atria and venous system behind it.[3] Some 80 years later, the forward theory related the clinical manifestations of heart failure to inadequate delivery of blood to the arterial system.[4] Although backward and forward heart failure can occur in isolation, for example in pulmonary embolism and cardiogenic shock, respectively, it no longer seems fruitful to make a rigid distinction between them as both are observed in the vast majority of patients.[1]

> The distinction between forward and backward failure arose as a result of efforts to explain the symptoms and signs of heart failure

Chronic heart failure

Chronic heart failure is the most common manifestation of heart failure, and the one with which this publication is principally concerned. The term has largely replaced expressions such as congestive cardiac failure, left heart failure, left ventricular failure and low-output failure, as it describes more accurately the persistent nature of the condition.

Chronic heart failure often follows an undulating course punctuated by acute exacerbations (so-called decompensated chronic heart failure) that require hospital admission. It occurs when the same anatomical abnormalities which cause acute heart failure develop gradually, or when the patient survives the initial insult as a result of a number of adaptive mechanisms, but has depressed cardiac function either at rest or on effort.

Ideally, the clinical syndrome of chronic heart failure should be diagnosed when first, a patient has symptoms of heart failure at rest or on effort, and second, he or she has objective evidence of cardiac dysfunction at rest.

Observation of a response to treatment with a diuretic, digoxin or an angiotensin-converting enzyme (ACE) inhibitor is also desirable, particularly when the diagnosis is in doubt.[5]

No simpler or more objective definition is currently available because no cut-off value of cardiac dysfunction, whether in terms of contraction, flow, pressure, dimension or volume, can be used reliably to identify subjects with heart failure. At present, the diagnosis therefore relies on good clinical judgement based on the history, physical examination and appropriate investigations. Importantly, the diagnosis underlying the syndrome must always be sought so that optimum treatment can be provided.

> The diagnosis underlying chronic heart failure must always be sought so that optimum treatment can be provided

Cardiac dysfunction

Cardiac dysfunction is an essential element in the diagnosis of heart failure, and many types can lead to the chronic syndrome. Valvular, endocardial, pericardial and myocardial pathologies are all capable of producing the end-stage condition of dyspnoea, fatigue and fluid retention. The relative contributions of each vary geographically with the prevalence of the important types of heart disease, i.e. ischaemic, hypertensive, rheumatic, valvular, infective, congenital and cardiomyopathic.

Left ventricular dysfunction

By far the commonest cause of chronic heart failure in industrialized societies is myocardial disease due to left ventricular dysfunction, particularly left ventricular systolic dysfunction. In this condition, pump failure occurs as a consequence of failed contraction of the left ventricle, most often as a result of myocardial loss secondary to myocardial infarction.

Less commonly, chronic heart failure can result from diastolic dysfunction, in which failed relaxation of the left ventricle in diastole leads to impaired filling. Diastolic dysfunction accounts for 30–40% of all chronic heart failure, becomes increasingly prevalent with advancing age, and is more common in individuals with pre-existing systemic hypertension.[6, 7] In addition, it is the predominant variety of ventricular dysfunction in rarer conditions such as hypertrophic obstructive cardiomyopathy and amyloid.

The natural history of diastolic dysfunction is not well-studied, but the condition is known to be associated with a better prognosis than systolic dysfunction.[8] The diagnostic distinction between diastolic and systolic dysfunction is important, as their treatments differ.

In patients with left ventricular dysfunction due to atherosclerosis, the picture is complicated by the fact that systolic and diastolic dysfunction often coexist: the former due to loss of myocardium and the latter due to the replacement of lost muscle by less compliant fibrous tissue.

> In patients with left ventricular dysfunction due to atherosclerosis, the picture is complicated by the fact that systolic and diastolic dysfunction often coexist

Left ventricular systolic dysfunction

Chronic heart failure is now thought to lie at the end-stage of a progressive deterioration in left ventricular function which can remain asymptomatic for years. In other words, when doctors diagnose heart failure by symptoms and signs, they are detecting a condition that, untreated, may have a mortality of up to 50% per annum.[9] The full-blown syndrome can be preceded by a long latent phase in which diagnosis on clinical grounds is impossible, but when left ventricular damage is certainly present. This state is commonly referred to as asymptomatic left ventricular dysfunction.

> When doctors diagnose heart failure on symptoms and signs, they are detecting a condition that, untreated, may have a mortality of up to 50% per annum

Natural history of left ventricular dysfunction

When the Framingham heart study first reported its epidemiological findings, on a cohort of subjects recruited in 1949, hypertension accounted for 75% of all the heart failure identified.[10] Recent evidence has confirmed that coronary artery disease accounts for the significant majority (between two-thirds and three-quarters) of cases of chronic heart failure.[11] For most people, therefore, the sequence of events begins at the time of an acute myocardial infarction.

In the Framingham study, 15% of patients with acute myocardial infarction went on to develop chronic heart failure over a 5-year period.[12, 13] However, those findings predated the widespread use of thrombolytic therapy and aspirin, as a result of which many more patients now survive acute myocardial infarction.[14] Research in the post thrombolytic era has shown that heart failure occurs, at least transiently, in 35% of patients admitted to hospital with acute myocardial infarction.[15]

Although many patients develop transient left ventricular failure in the acute phase of myocardial infarction, most recover satisfactorily (despite electrocardiographic and cardiac enzyme evidence of substantial myocardial damage), to be left with asymptomatic left ventricular dysfunction. In this state, symptoms and signs of heart failure are lacking, but objective measurement of indices of global left ventricular systolic function (either non-invasively by echocardiography or radionuclide ventriculography, or invasively by angiocardiography) reveals depressed left ventricular contractility. Normally, the left ventricular ejection fraction is quoted as the parameter with which to express left ventricular systolic dysfunction, as it is associated independently with prognosis.[16] The cut-off value taken to indicate significant left ventricular systolic dysfunction varies with the method of measurement and between centres, but is generally 35–40%.

> Heart failure occurs, at least transiently, in 35% of patients admitted to hospital with acute myocardial infarction

Information on the prevalence of left ventricular dysfunction post-infarction is scarce other than in highly selected patients randomized in clinical trials. One of the largest post myocardial infarction ACE inhibitor trials, the Survival and Ventricular Enlargement (SAVE) trial, found that 40% of myocardial infarction survivors had objective evidence of left ventricular dysfunction in the form of a left ventricular ejection fraction of ≤40% (by radionuclide ventriculography); 14% had symptomatic left ventricular dysfunction, i.e. chronic heart failure, and 25% were left with asymptomatic left ventricular dysfunction.[17]

What subsequently happens to these post myocardial infarction patients with asymptomatic left ventricular dysfunction is not well-documented. Some develop recurrent myocardial infarction, which further compromises their left ventricular function and tips them into overt chronic heart failure (Fig. 1.1). Others, however, progress to the heart failure stage without further myocardial infarction. The heart appears to undergo a process of remodelling resulting in progressive loss of contractile function leading to symptomatic left ventricular dysfunction. In these subjects, the initial infarct size is possibly the dominant factor in their progression to overt heart failure.[18] Other contributing risk factors are the neuroendocrine, vascular and renal responses that occur in individuals with left ventricular dysfunction.

Although all would appear to be well in subjects with asymptomatic left ventricular dysfunction, there is evidence to

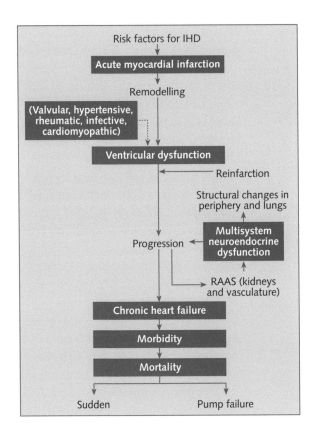

FIG. 1.1 From myocardial infarction to chronic heart failure. IHD = ischaemic heart disease; RAAS = renin–angiotensin–aldosterone system.

suggest that compensatory neuroendocrine activation is already occurring: noradrenaline is elevated,[19] as is N-terminal atrial natriuretic peptide.[20] In addition, impairment of aerobic capacity on exercise has been demonstrated.[21]

Multisystem dysfunction

The primary problem in chronic heart failure is cardiac, but the clinical syndrome is characterized by secondary multisystem dysfunction which ultimately leads to a terminal state of multiorgan failure.

> The primary problem in chronic heart failure is cardiac, but the clinical syndrome is characterized by secondary multisystem dysfunction

Returning to the physiological definition of heart failure, blood pressure is an important contributor to the adequacy of oxygenation of metabolizing tissues,[22] and cardiac output is a major determinant of the blood pressure. The reduction in cardiac output which occurs in left ventricular dysfunction activates a myriad of mechanisms which, presumably, were designed to protect the organism from haemorrhage.

Briefly, the sympathetic nervous system is activated and adrenaline released, resulting in an increased heart rate and vasoconstriction. A decrease in renal perfusion results in activation of the renin–angiotensin–aldosterone system, leading to production of the powerful vasoconstrictor angiotensin II and, ultimately, sodium retention through the actions of aldosterone. Water retention is also augmented by vasopressin production from the posterior pituitary. Other potent vasoconstrictors such as endothelin contribute to the increase in peripheral vascular resistance. These changes may not be sufficiently counteracted by the cardiac endocrine system which produces the natriuretic and vasodilating atrial and brain natriuretic peptides; as a result, the syndrome of heart failure supervenes in many patients.

Ultimately, as a consequence of this extensive compensatory activity, structural changes take place in the vascular arterioles, leading to increasing stiffness of the vessels. In addition, morphological changes occur in skeletal muscle, and respiratory function is affected by an increase in physiological dead space and airways obstruction. This vicious circle does not help the heart, which remodels and dilates further with a consequent reduction in cardiac output, electrical instability and thrombus formation which will ultimately lead to death either from progressive pump failure or suddenly as a result of arrhythmia.

> As a consequence of extensive compensatory activity, structural changes take place in the vascular arterioles, leading to increasing stiffness of the vessels

Concluding definition

In keeping with the growing awareness that chronic heart failure is not just an isolated cardiac response to a wide range of insults, but is a condition with numerous metabolic and endocrine effects, a more suitable definition for the clinician may be encompassed in the remarks by Packer: chronic heart failure represents a complex clinical syndrome characterized by abnormalities of left ventricular function and neurohormonal regulation which are accompanied by effort intolerance, fluid retention and reduced longevity.[23]

> Chronic heart failure is not just an isolated cardiac response to a wide range of insults, but is a condition with numerous metabolic and endocrine effects

References

1 Braunwald E, Grossman W. Clinical aspects of heart failure. In: Braunwald E (ed) *Heart Disease*, 4th edn. WB Saunders, New York. 1992; 444.

2 Lenfant C. Report of the task force on research in heart failure. *Circulation* 1994; **90**: 1118–1123.

3 Hope JA. *Treatise on the Diseases of the Heart and Great Vessels*. William-Kidd, London, 1832.

4 Mackenzie J. *Diseases of the Heart*, 3rd edn. Oxford University Press, London, 1913.

5 The Task Force on Heart Failure of the European Society of Cardiology. Guidelines for the diagnosis of heart failure. *Eur Heart Journal* 1995; **16**: 741–751.

6 Dougherty AH, Naccarelli GV, Gray EL, Hicks CH, Goldstein RA. Congestive heart failure with normal systolic function. *Am J Cardiol* 1984; **54**: 778–782.

7 Soufer R, Wohlgelertner D, Vita NA *et al*. Intact systolic left ventricular function in clinical congestive heart failure. *Am J Cardiol* 1985; **55**: 1032–1036.

8 Cohn JW, Johnson GJ and the Veterans Administration Cooperative Study Group. The Ve-HeFT study. *Circulation* 1990; **81**(suppl III): 11148–11153.

9 The CONSENSUS Trial Study Group. Effects of enalapril on mortality in severe congestive cardiac failure. *N Engl J Med* 1987; **316**: 1429–1435.

10 McKee PA, Castelli WP, McNamara PM, Kannel WB. The natural history of

congestive heart failure. *N Engl J Med* 1971; **285**: 781–787.

11 Teerlink JR, Goldhaber SZ, Pfeffer MA. An overview of contemporary etiologies of congestive heart failure. *Am Heart J* 1991; **121**: 1852–1853.

12 Kannel WB, Sorlie P, McNamara PM. Prognosis after initial myocardial infarction: the Framingham study. *Am J Cardiol* 1979; **44**: 53–59.

13 Kannel WB. Epidemiology and prevention of cardiac failure: Framingham study insights. *Eur Heart J* 1987; suppl F: 23–26.

14 Yusuf S. Wittes J, Friedman L. Overview of results of randomized clinical trials in heart disease. 1 Treatments following myocardial infarction. *JAMA* 1988; **260**: 2088–2093.

15 Stevenson R, Ranjadayalan K, Wilkinson P, Roberts R, Timmis AD. Short and long-term prognosis of acute myocardial infarction since the introduction of thrombolysis. *Br Med J* 1993; **307**: 349–353.

16 Nelson NB, Cohn PF, Garlin R. Prognosis in medically treated coronary artery disease. Influence of ejection fraction compared to other parameters. *Circulation* 1975; **52**: 408.

17 Pfeffer MA, Braunwald E, Moye LA *et al.* Effect of captopril on mortality in patients with left ventricular dysfunction after myocardial infarction. Results of the Survival and Ventricular Enlargement Trial. *N Engl J Med* 1992; **327**: 669–677.

18 Moye LA, Pfeffer MA, Braunwald E. Rationale, design and baseline characteristics of the survival and ventricular enlargement trial. *Am J Cardiol* 1989; **68**: 70D–79D.

19 Harris P. Congestive heart failure: central role of the arterial blood pressure. *Br Heart J* 1987; **58**: 190–203.

20 Francis G, Benedict C, Johnstone DE *et al.* Comparison of neuroendocrine activation in patients with left ventricular dysfunction with and without congestive heart failure: a substudy of the Studies of Left Ventricular Dysfunction (SOLVD). *Circulation* 1990; **82**: 1724–1729.

21 Lerman A, Gibbons RJ, Rodeheffer RJ *et al.* Circulating N terminal atrial natriuretic peptide as a marker for symptomless left ventricular dysfunction. *Lancet* 1993; **341**: 1105–1109.

22 Le Jemtel TH, Chang-seng L, Stewart DK *et al.* Reduced peak aerobic capacity in ventricular systolic dysfunction. *Circulation* 1994; **90**: 2757–2760.

23 Packer M. Survival in patients with chronic heart failure and its potential modification by drug therapy. In: Conh J (ed) *Drug Treatment of Heart Failure*, 2nd edn. ATC International, Secaucus, NJ. 1988; 273.

The Clinical Causes of Heart Failure

SUMMARY POINTS

- Abnormalities of the muscle, rhythm, valve or pericardium are all possible causes of chronic heart failure
- The majority of heart failure patients have myocardial dysfunction which is linked to coronary heart disease. More rarely myocardial dysfunction occurs in the presence of normal coronary vessels when the heart disease is termed cardiomyopathy
- Coronary heart disease can precipitate heart failure as a consequence of myocardial infarction, left ventricular aneurysm, multiple minor ischaemic events or apparent global inactivity of the myocardium
- Cardiomyopathy can be described as dilated, hypertrophic or restrictive and can be caused by toxins, infection, autoimmunity or a genetic predisposition
- Failure of the myocardium to relax in diastole is a common cause of heart failure in the elderly

Chronic heart failure has two major components: an abnormality of the heart itself, and the response of the body to the diminished ability of the heart to function as a pump. The symptoms and signs are largely a consequence of the long-term responses in the body. For example, the salt and water retention, common in chronic heart failure, are the result of abnormal function of the kidney, and the symptoms of shortness of breath and fatigue are related to chronic changes in skeletal muscle.[1] In contrast, the signs and symptoms in patients with acute heart failure are dominated by the haemodynamic consequences of the reduced performance of the heart as a pump.

The various descriptive terms for heart failure, such as forward, backward, low-flow, high-flow, right, left, overt, compensated, symptomatic and asymptomatic, may help doctors communicate, but do not advance our understanding of the physiology or underlying causes of heart failure. For practical

> Chronic heart failure has two major components: an abnormality of the heart, and the response of the body to the diminished ability of the heart to function as a pump

purposes, heart failure can usefully be classified as acute heart failure, chronic heart failure or circulatory shock. Acute heart failure is synonymous with pulmonary oedema. Chronic heart failure is a persistent syndrome of which sodium and water retention is a common feature and almost the hallmark. Circulatory shock is characterized by low blood pressure, oliguria or anuria, and a cold constricted periphery.

Chronic heart failure

Chronic heart failure resulting from diminished function of the heart as a pump is invariably caused by an abnormality of the muscle, rhythm, valves or pericardium (Table 2.1).

TABLE 2.1 Causes of heart failure.
Myocardial disease
Arrhythmias
Valve disease
Pericardial disease
Congenital heart disease

Abnormalities of the myocardium are by far the commonest reason for heart failure. Myocardial failure has traditionally been divided into myocardial abnormalities due to coronary heart disease, accounting for almost 80%, and those which occur due to an abnormality of the myocardium in the presence of normal coronary arteries (cardiomyopathy). Coronary angiography is necessary to distinguish between the two.

> Abnormalities of the myocardium are by far the most common cause of heart failure

Myocardial failure due to coronary heart disease

Myocardial failure due to coronary heart disease includes a number of pathological states (Table 2.2). Most common is a reduction in the total number of functioning myocytes due to acute myocardial infarction. More subtle abnormalities include left ventricular aneurysm, multiple minor ischaemic events or apparent global inactivity of the myocardium in the presence of extensive three-vessel coronary heart disease (hibernation). An additional, but often overlooked, cause of heart failure is the poorly coordinated contraction of the left ventricle common in coronary heart disease.

TABLE 2.2 Causes of heart failure due to myocardial disease.	
Systolic failure	
Coronary artery disease	Local dyskinesia
	Diffuse dysfunction
	Incoordination
	Aneurysm
	Stunning or hibernation
Cardiomyopathy	*Dilated*
	Idiopathic dilated cardiomyopathy
	Genetic and/or sporadic origin
	Familial
	Alcohol
	Myocarditis, viruses, infectious agents, autoimmunity
	Heavy metals, toxins and poisons
	Adriamycin and other cardiotoxic drugs
	Collagen disorders
	Neuromuscular disorders
	Peripartum cardiomyopathy
	Metabolic disorders
	Hypertrophic (HCM and ASH)
	Familial
	Genetic and sporadic
	Restrictive
	Amyloid, sarcoid, haemochromatosis
	Endocardial fibrosis
Hypertension	
Drugs	β-Blockers
	Calcium antagonists
	Antiarrhythmic drugs
Diastolic failure	
Elderly	
Ischaemia	
Hypertrophy	

HCM, Hypertrophic cardiomyopathy; ASH, asymmetric septal hypertrophy.

Several other entities have been recently described as occurring with coronary heart disease (Table 2.3): stunning is mechanical dysfunction that persists after reperfusion in the absence of irreversible damage and despite restoration of normal or near-normal coronary flow.[2] Diminished contraction of the myocardium can continue for up to 24 h despite the restoration of normal blood flow. Hibernation is a state of persistently impaired myocardial and left ventricular function at rest due to reduced coronary blood flow. It can be partially or completely restored to normal if the myocardial oxygen supply/demand relationship is favourably altered by improving blood flow and/or by reducing demand.[3] The blood flow reduction is not sufficient to cause the death of the myocyte, but brings about metabolic changes that diminish its ability to contract. The latter syndrome is receiving increasing attention as measures taken to increase blood flow, including coronary artery bypass surgery and percutaneous angioplasty, might have a therapeutic advantage.

TABLE 2.3 Modish terms and concepts in coronary heart disease.
Stunning
Hibernation
Mummified myocardium
Stuttering ischaemia
Preconditioning
Remodelling
Chronic ischaemia
Ischaemic cardiomyopathy

Other recently described entities include stuttering ischaemia and preconditioning. Preconditioning is the phenomenon whereby the ability of the myocardium to recover after a period of ischaemia is enhanced by a previous short period of ischaemia. Remodelling refers to shape changes that occur after myocardial infarction or during exacerbations of heart failure. Enlargement of the heart is an active metabolic process and amenable to modification by drugs which do not simply affect fluid retention or central haemodynamics.

> Enlargement of the heart is an active metabolic process and amenable to drugs which do not simply affect fluid retention or central haemodynamics

Cardiomyopathies

Cardiomyopathies are diseases of the myocardium leading to abnormal cardiac function in the absence of coronary heart disease, hypertension, congenital distortion, valve or pericardial disease. They have traditionally been classified into three types:

1   Hypertrophic.
2   Restrictive.
3   Dilated (formerly congestive).

The three syndromes are distinguished by physiological, anatomical and clinical features (Table 2.2), but are not entirely exclusive.

Dilated cardiomyopathy

Dilated cardiomyopathy (DCM) is characterized by an enlarged ventricle and an ejection fraction <45% or M-mode fractional shortening <30%. Significant coronary heart disease (as indicated by symptoms, evidence of ischaemia or a stenosis >50% on a coronary angiogram) must be excluded. Hypertension, valve disease, pericardial disease, acute myocarditis and arrhythmias should not be present.

Studies in Denmark, Sweden, the UK and the USA report the incidence of DCM in the community to be between 5 and 10 per 100 000 of the population. The prevalence is 40 per 100 000. More men than women are affected and the condition is 2.5 times more common in Blacks than Caucasians after taking account of potential confounders such as alcohol intake, body size and income. The prevalence of all types of heart failure in the community is approximately 1–2% and the incidence about 0.4%.

> The prevalence of heart failure in the community is approximately 1–2% and the incidence about 0.4%. Four per cent of patients have heart failure due to DCM

DCM is by far the most common clinically detected cardiomyopathy, accounting for about 4% of patients with heart failure in the community. Higher figures are reported in large trials because those patients have been selected from hospital admissions.

Aetiology

Approximately 25% of DCM are familial and may have a specific cause which is yet to be defined. About 70% are idiopathic. The major putative mechanisms for idiopathic DCM are:
- viral infection (enteroviruses, Coxsackie B, influenza virus, and mumps);
- toxins

- immunological mechanisms;
- genetic disorders.

An initial infection or insult to the myocardium may initiate a series of biological events that leads to a chronic condition.

In a recently reported hospital series of 673 consecutive unselected cases of DCM, 47% were diagnosed as idiopathic DCM, 12% as idiopathic myocarditis, 11% as coronary artery disease, 5% each as human immunodeficiency virus (HIV) or peripartum, 3% each as alcoholic or drug-induced cardiomyopathy, and 2% as connective tissue disease, hypertension, amyloidosis or familial cardiomyopathy.[4] Thus, the commonest cause of DCM is unknown.

Excessive alcohol intake is a common identifiable cause of DCM, although the precise incidence varies with the population being studied. Ten per cent of alcoholics have manifestations of cardiomyopathy. Liver cirrhosis is not particularly predictive.

> Ten per cent of alcoholics have manifestations of cardiomyopathy

Alcohol abuse leads to cardiomyopathy in three distinct ways. The acute toxic effect may lead to acute heart failure or heart failure brought on by an arrhythmia, commonly atrial fibrillation. Long-term intake leads to chronic DCM which may present as chronic heart failure or heart failure due to an arrhythmia. The third presentation is as part of a general nutritional deficiency. In particular, alcohol abuse is associated with thiamine deficiency (beriberi). Another presentation occurs as a consequence of toxic substances in the alcoholic beverage. For example, an outbreak of cardiomyopathy in Canada was eventually attributed to excessive cobalt in beer.

Alcoholic cardiomyopathy is related to the degree of consumption and is common in individuals who consume 80 g/day or more or who have a lifetime consumption of more than 250 kg (one standard unit of spirits or a glass of wine contains 10 g of alcohol). There is great variation in the severity of the cardiac effects of alcohol. The diagnosis is usually suspected from a careful history, but patients are often reluctant to admit to a high alcohol intake or underestimate how much they drink.

Hypertrophic cardiomyopathy

Hypertrophic cardiomyopathy (HCM) is characterized by a hypertrophied and non-dilated left and/or right ventricle in the absence of a cardiac or systemic cause. The myocardium shows disarray of hypertrophied and disorganized myocytes, and increased thickness; identical histological abnormalities have recently been reported when myocardial thickening was absent. The hypertrophy is often in the septum (asymmetric septal hypertrophy or ASH), but can extend throughout the ventricle or be localized to the apex. In some cases, premature contraction of the mid-portion of the ventricle results in a systolic gradient and outflow obstruction known as hypertrophic obstructive cardiomyopathy (HOCM). HCM is rare, but can run in families and is associated with sudden death. A genetic defect can be detected in as many as 60% of cases. HCM should be distinguished from athletic heart, a common but benign condition in which substantial reversible hypertrophy of the ventricle can occur.

Restrictive cardiomyopathy

This is a very rare condition characterized by a stiff ventricle which is not greatly enlarged; the hallmark is abnormal diastolic function which limits ventricular filling. The most common causes are amyloidosis and endocardial fibrosis.

Diastolic heart failure

In recent years, much attention has been paid to diastolic heart failure (Table 2.4), or malfunction of the heart due to inability of the ventricle to fill appropriately in diastole. A simple example is severe mitral stenosis in which, because of the obstruction to the valve, blood cannot enter the ventricle quickly enough during a short diastole.

TABLE 2.4 Diastolic heart failure.
Heart failure with a near-normal-sized heart and normal ejection fraction at rest
Failure of the ventricle to fill at end-diastole
Common in community, not hospital practice
Common in elderly, hypertensives and those with coronary heart disease
Often presents with breathlessness and fatigue
Difficult to treat

Diastolic heart failure due to an inability of the ventricular muscle to relax often occurs in patients who have a normal-sized heart. It is commonly assumed that a normal-sized ventricle must have normal systolic function, but the size of the ventricle is not a good measure of its function in systole. In practice, most patients with diastolic heart failure also have systolic heart failure. The findings may be dominated by abnormalities of relaxation, but exercise systolic contraction is also abnormal. In order to be certain a patient has diastolic heart failure it is necessary to show abnormal filling of the left ventricle on exercise when symptoms occur, and normal systolic function. Unfortunately, accurate measurement of the end-diastolic volume of the left ventricle on exercise is difficult, if not impossible.

> It is assumed that a normal-sized ventricle must have normal systolic function, but the size of the ventricle is not a good measure of its function in systole

In hospital studies, the prevalence of diastolic heart failure is low and only accounts for approximately 5–10% of patients. In the community, the prevalence may be higher because many patients have only minor symptoms and are never hospitalized. It has been claimed that 50% of patients with heart failure have diastolic heart failure.[5] The significance of this figure depends critically on how heart failure was diagnosed and on the population from which the patients were drawn.

One particularly common form of diastolic heart failure occurs in the elderly. The total number of myocytes is often reduced and the remainder are hypertrophied. The ventricle is fibrosed, and coronary heart disease or hypertension is often present. The result is a heart which is not greatly enlarged, but has thickened myocardium and relaxes poorly. Salt and water retention do not usually dominate the clinical picture. The patient feels tired and is short of breath on exercise. Treatment is particularly difficult, but the prognosis is better than that seen in heart failure with an enlarged heart.[6]

Hypertensive heart failure

The extent to which hypertension is a cause of heart failure is disputed. High blood pressure is a powerful risk factor for coronary heart disease, and much of the association may be as a result of the progression of atheroma and the occurrence of ischaemic events, rather than a consequence of hypertension itself. In the Framingham study, hypertension was a cause of heart failure in up to 70% of cases.[7, 8] More recent studies have reported a figure of no more than 10%.[9, 10] The difference may be partly a matter of classification. What is certain is that hypertension is a risk factor for the progression of heart failure and is a powerful exacerbating factor. Hypertension not only increases the work of the heart, but also increases the likelihood of coronary events.

> Hypertension not only increases the work of the heart, but also increases the likelihood of coronary events

Valve disorders

That abnormalities of the cardiac valves now rarely cause heart failure is largely because of the decline in the incidence of rheumatic fever. Aortic stenosis in the elderly can easily be overlooked as a cause of heart failure and appears to be becoming more prevalent.

Acute heart failure

Acute heart failure is a clinical syndrome in which a sudden and rapid deterioration of the ability of the heart to eject blood results in acute pulmonary oedema. By far the commonest cause is acute myocardial infarction, but other causes include the onset of an acute arrhythmia or rupture of a papillary muscle resulting in acute mitral regurgitation. Most conditions that cause chronic heart failure can also give rise to acute heart failure. Usually there is some precipitating condition. Importantly, acute heart failure must be distinguished from the many other causes of rapid-onset of shortness of breath, such as a pneumothorax, massive pulmonary embolus, asthma and lung disease.

> Acute heart failure must be distinguished from the many other causes for rapid-onset of shortness of breath

Admissions to hospital

Patients frequently present in casualty with the syndrome of overt heart failure. The reasons for the presentation or admission to hospital may differ substantially from the causes of heart failure.

Some of the causes of worsening myocardial function are shown in Table 2.5. Table 2.6 lists the causes of readmission or deterioration in patients with heart failure. Data on this practical problem are hard to obtain. There is a need for comprehensive population-based studies (Table 2.7). Furthermore, the type of evidence often presented relates to the risk factors for heart failure (dominated by coronary heart disease) and prognostic factors, rather than the causes of the acute exacerbation (Table 2.8).

TABLE 2.5 Causes of worsening myocardial function.

Ischaemic event, hibernation or stunning
Exposure to toxic agent
   Alcohol
   Viruses
   Drugs
Cell morphology and orientation — hypertrophy
Altered haemodynamics
   Hypertension
   Valve function
Apoptosis

TABLE 2.6 Causes of readmission or deterioration in patients with heart failure.

Myocardial infarction or ischaemic episode
Arrhythmia
Pulmonary or systemic oedema
Dietary indiscretion
Non-compliance with medicines
Adverse drug-related event
Exposure to toxic agent
Stroke
Synergistic medical problem
Non-cardiovascular event
Social circumstances
Reassessment of medicines

In a district hospital, pulmonary oedema and arrhythmias were the most frequent causes of admission.[11] The most common aetiology was coronary heart disease, but a precise diagnosis was not possible in many patients because coronary angiography was not routinely performed and the diagnosis of coronary heart disease could only be made with certainty on the basis of other indicators in 41% (Table 2.9).[12] Up to 53% of readmissions of elderly patients may be preventable and are related more to social and organizational matters than the medical diagnosis (Table 2.10).[11] From the practical point of view, much can be done to help patients with heart failure by paying attention to detail. Many of the reasons for admission to hospital can be treated and the hospital admission avoided.

> From the practical point of view, much can be done to help patients with heart failure by paying attention to detail

TABLE 2.7 Sources of data on progression of heart failure.

Population-based studies
Physician records
Hospital records for admissions and discharges
Controlled trials

TABLE 2.8 Types of data on progression of heart failure.

Risk factors
Similar to those for coronary heart disease

Prognostic factors	
Heart size	Ejection fraction
Ventricular function	Peak MVO$_2$
Metabolic markers	Plasma sodium, atrial natriuretic
	factor, noradrenaline

Acute causes

TABLE 2.9 Admissions with heart failure to a district general hospital.

Presentation	%	Aetiology	%
Pulmonary oedema	51	Coronary heart disease	41
Pulmonary oedema			
+ myocardial infarction	11	Valve disease	9.3
Fluid overload	38	Hypertension	6.4
		Cor pulmonale	2.9
Arrhythmia	37	Cardiomyopathy	1.4
		Congenital	1.4
		Thyrotoxicosis	1.4
		Unknown	36.4

Population of 155 000. In 6 months 2877 admissions, 140 (4.9%) with heart failure: 51% male; 73 years.
From Parameshwar *et al.*[12] with permission.

TABLE 2.10 Readmission of elderly patients with heart failure.	
161 hospitalized patients over 70 years in St Louis, USA	
Hospital mortality 13%, 47% readmitted within 90 days	
Recurrent heart failure	57%
Other cardiac conditions	8%
Non-cardiac illness	32%
Of readmissions 53% probably preventable	
Non-compliance drugs	15%
Non-compliance diet	18%
Inadequate discharge plan	15%
Inadequate follow-up	20%
Failed social support	21%
Failure to seek help	20%

From Vinson et al.[11] with permission.

References

1 Coats AJS, Clark AL, Piepoli M, Volterrani M, Poole-Wilson PA. Symptoms and quality of life in heart failure: the muscle hypothesis. *Br Heart J* 1994; **72**: 36–43.

2 Bolli R. Mechanism of myocardial 'stunning'. *Circulation* 1990; **82**: 723–738.

3 Rahimtoola SH. A perspective on the three large multicenter randomised clinical trials of coronary bypass surgery for chronic stable angina. *Circulation* 1985; **72**: V123–V135.

4 Kasper EK, Agema WRP, Hutchins GM, Deckers JW, Hare JM, Baughman KL. The causes of dilated cardiomyopathy: a clinicopathologic review of 673 consecutive patients. *J Am Coll Cardiol* 1924; **23**: 586–590.

5 Dougherty AH, Naccarelli GV, Gray EL, Hicks CH, Goldstein RA. Congestive heart failure with normal systolic function. *Am J Cardiol* 1984; **54**: 778–782.

6 Brogan WC, Hillis LD, Flores ED, Lange RA. The natural history of isolated left ventricular diastolic dysfunction. *Am J Med* 1992; **92**: 627–630.

7 McKee PA, Castelli WP, McNamara PM, Kannel WB. The natural history of congestive heart failure: the Framingham study. *N Engl J Med* 1971; **285**: 1441–1446.

8 Kannel WB, Belanger JA. Epidemiology of heart failure. *Am Heart J* 1991; **121**: 951–956.

9 Teerlink JR, Goldhaber SZ, Pfeffer MA. An overview of contemporary aetiologies of congestive heart failure. *Am Heart J* 1991; **121**: 1852–1853.

10 Parameshwar J, Shackell MM, Richardson A, Poole-Wilson PA, Sutton GC. Prevalence of heart failure in three general practices in north west London. *J Gen Practic* 1992; **42**: 287–289.

11 Vinson JM, Rich MW, Sperry JC, Shah AS, McNamara T. Early readmission of elderly patients with congestive heart failure. *J Am Geriatr Soc* 1992; **38**: 1290–1295.

12 Parameshwar J, Poole-Wilson PA, Sutton GC. Heart failure in a district hospital. *J R Coll Phys* 1992; **26**: 139–142.

The Public Health Problem of Heart Failure

SUMMARY POINTS

- Epidemiological surveys indicate that heart failure affects between 1 and 2% of the population in Europe and the USA
- The prevalence of heart failure increases sharply with age, affecting perhaps as many as 10% of individuals over the age of 80
- Mortality from heart failure correlates with disease severity. Annual mortality exceeds 60% in severe cases, but even in milder forms, approximately half of patients die within 5 years of diagnosis
- There is a high incidence of sudden cardiac death in patients with heart failure
- The high utilization of health care resources by patients with heart failure places a considerable economic burden on health care systems

Despite an overall decline in total cardiovascular disease mortality in industrialized countries over the last two decades,[1] chronic heart failure continues to represent a major and escalating health care problem. The precise medical and socioeconomic consequences of heart failure are difficult to quantify, largely because of the lack of a universally accepted definition and its protean clinical manifestations. Urgent efforts are therefore required to improve our understanding of its causes and pathophysiological mechanisms in order to develop more effective treatment modalities and, perhaps more importantly, preventive strategies.

Chronic heart failure continues to represent a major and escalating health care problem

Epidemiology

Reliable epidemiological data about the occurrence of heart failure in the general population are scarce. The core problem is that there are no agreed criteria by which a definite diagnosis can be established. However, surveys indicate that heart failure affects 1–2% of the population in Europe and the USA. The prevalence increases sharply with age, affecting perhaps as many as 10% of individuals over the age of 80 years.

Both incidence and prevalence appear to be rising steeply, probably due mainly to the ageing of the population and recent improvements in the medical management of acute myocardial infarction. The net effect of these various demographic trends is that the heart failure epidemic is likely to continue to escalate into the next century; it has been estimated that there will be a 30% increase in the number of very elderly people over the course of the next decade[2] and consequently that the prevalence of heart failure may increase by as much as 70% by the year 2010.[3]

> The prevalence of heart failure may increase by as much as 70% by the year 2010

Ischaemic heart disease appears to have superseded hypertension as the principal cause of heart failure. However, it can be difficult to establish which is the primary cause because hypertension and coronary artery disease are pathophysiologically linked and often coexist in the same individual.

Morbidity

Although ventricular dysfunction may be asymptomatic, heart failure is associated with a high symptom burden in the vast majority of patients and results in greater impairment of quality of life than any other chronic medical illness. A study of the impact of various common medical disorders on patient-reported quality of life showed that heart failure had the greatest negative effect, by a substantial margin.[4] Quality of life is adversely affected, even in patients with mild-to-moderate heart failure. In the study of men born in 1913, patients with heart failure had more physical complaints, spent more time in bed, had less energy and were less fit than those without heart failure.[5]

A study of the impact of common medical disorders on patient-reported quality of life showed that heart failure had the greatest negative effect by a substantial margin

Not surprisingly, quality of life impairment correlates with disease severity; patients with more severe heart failure seek medical attention more frequently, consume more medication and are hospitalized more often than patients with milder disease.

In patients with cardiovascular disease, heart failure ranks second only to hypertension as a reason for an outpatient consultation.[6] In the UK, about 120 000 people (0.2% of the population) require hospitalization for heart failure each year.[7] This represents about 5% of all adult medical and geriatric admissions, and exceeds the number of patients admitted with myocardial infarction or unstable angina.[7, 8] Hospitalization is usually prolonged (average duration in the UK is about 11 days on an acute medical ward and 4 weeks on an acute geriatric ward) and frequently recurrent (about one-third of patients are readmitted within 12 months of discharge).[7, 8]

Collectively, these dismal statistics highlight the scale of the morbid burden imposed by heart failure. However, on a more positive note, several large placebo-controlled studies have clearly shown that modern vasodilator therapies, in particular angiotensin-converting enzyme (ACE) inhibitors, can improve symptoms and correspondingly reduce the frequency (and perhaps duration) of hospitalization in patients with heart failure. This will be discussed in more detail below.

Heart failure is associated with important cardiovascular comorbidity. In the Framingham study, individuals with heart failure had a fourfold increased risk of stroke (rivalling atrial fibrillation) and an up to fivefold increased risk of myocardial infarction compared with the general population.[9] It is important not to forget that heart failure (invariably a progressive and ultimately fatal illness) also imposes a significant morbid burden upon the relatives of sufferers.

Heart failure (invariably a progressive and ultimately fatal illness) also imposes a significant morbid burden upon the relatives of sufferers

Mortality

Despite significant recent advances in our understanding of its pathophysiological mechanisms and the associated development of novel therapeutic strategies, chronic heart failure remains a highly lethal condition with the sort of grim prognosis traditionally associated with malignant disease. The probability of dying within 5 years of diagnosis of heart failure in the original Framingham study cohort was 62% in men (a poorer prognosis than after a myocardial infarction) and 42% in women.[10] Forty-year Framingham follow-up data confirmed these prognostic trends, with 5-year survival rates of only 25% for men and 38% for women with heart failure.[11]

> The probability of dying within 5 years of diagnosis of heart failure in the original Framingham study cohort was 62% in men and 42% in women

The lethal nature of heart failure is highlighted by the fact that average 5-year survival for all cancers in men and women in the USA between 1979 and 1984 was about 50%.[12] Median survival following a diagnosis of heart failure in the Framingham cohort was only 1.7 years in men and 3.2 years in women.[11, 12]

Mortality from heart failure was determined 10 and 15 years after identification of the original study cohort in the National Health and Nutrition Examination Survey (NHANES), generating data more applicable to the general population than that derived from Framingham or any other observational study.[13] Ten-year mortality for individuals aged 25–74 years with self-reported heart failure was 50% for men and 43% for women. When heart failure was diagnosed according to a clinical scoring system, 10-year mortality was 54% for men and 38% for women. Fifteen-year mortalities (determined only for individuals aged 55–74 years) were 63% in men and 57% in women with self-reported heart failure; 72% of men and 56% of women with heart failure diagnosed according to clinical criteria died within 15 years of diagnosis. Mortality from heart failure increased with advancing age at the time of diagnosis.

The results of various other studies addressing mortality from heart failure in smaller population subgroups are less applicable to the general population, but have conveyed the same core message as the larger studies: prognosis is extremely poor once symptoms and clinical signs of heart failure are manifest, and the majority of patients die within 5 years of diagnosis.

> Prognosis is extremely poor once symptoms and clinical signs of heart failure are manifest, and the majority of patients die within 5 years of diagnosis

Mortality from heart failure increases with the clinical severity of the condition.[14] In CONSENSUS, 1-year mortality in patients with severe New York Heart Association (NYHA) class IV heart failure given placebo was a striking 63%.[15] Similarly, in Studies of Left Ventricular Dysfunction (SOLVD) the mortality for patients in the same class was 64% over the mean 41.4 month follow-up period, compared with 51%, 35% and 30% for those with class III, II and I disease, respectively.[16] Resting left ventricular ejection fraction is another powerful predictor of prognosis in patients with heart failure. In SOLVD, 50% of patients with ejection fractions between 6% and 22% died during follow-up, compared with only 28% of patients who had an ejection fraction between 30% and 35%.[16]

Given that neuroendocrine activation is most marked in those heart failure patients with most impaired ventricular function, it is logical that plasma renin activity and circulating levels of noradrenaline and atrial natriuretic peptide should also be powerful predictors of prognosis in SOLVD. Other clinical parameters associated with an adverse prognosis include:
- poor exercise tolerance;
- presence of atrial fibrillation;
- plasma electrolyte abnormalities (especially hyponatraemia);
- coronary artery disease as the underlying aetiology of heart failure.

Many patients who die from heart failure do so as a result of sudden cardiac death rather than progressive pump failure. The mechanism is controversial, but ventricular tachydysrhythmias are probably the primary cause. Although it is widely accepted that ACE inhibitors delay progression of heart failure, their effect on the incidence of sudden death remains controversial.

> Many patients who die from heart failure do so as a result of sudden cardiac death rather than progressive pump failure

Costs

Heart failure is an extremely costly illness in terms of the morbidity it causes in individual patients (and their families) and the high utilization of health care resources that follows. Several recent economic analyses have consistently shown heart failure to account for between 1% and 2% of total spending on health care in Europe and the USA (Table 3.1).[6,17–19] In the UK, the direct cost to the National Health Service (NHS) has been estimated at £360 million per year.[18] This is equivalent to about 1.2% of total annual NHS expenditure, about 10% of annual spending on diseases of the circulatory system, and is similar to the direct costs of asthma. In the USA, expenditure on heart failure is comparable with that on hypertension, but is about fivefold greater than spending on lung cancer.[6]

Heart failure accounts for between 1% and 2% of total spending on health care in Europe and the USA

TABLE 3.1 In the Framingham study, two major or one major and two minor criteria had to be present concurrently to establish a diagnosis of heart failure. Minor criteria were only satisfied if they could not be attributed to another medical condition.

Major criteria	Minor criteria
Paroxysmal nocturnal dyspnoea or orthopnoea	Bilateral ankle oedema
Neck vein distension	Nocturnal cough
Rales	Dyspnoea on exertion
Radiographic cardiomegaly	Hepatomegaly
Acute pulmonary oedema	Pleural effusion
Third heart sound/gallop rhythm	Vital capacity reduced by
Increased central venous pressure (>16 cm water)	a third from maximum
Circulation time ≥25 s	Tachycardia ≥120
Hepatojugular reflux	beats/min
Pulmonary oedema, visceral congestion or cardiomegaly at autopsy	

An additional major *or* minor criterion was weight loss of ≥4.5kg in 5 days in response to treatment.

Hospital admissions are a major constituent of the economic costs of any chronic illness. In heart failure, hospitalization has been estimated to account for a remarkable two-thirds of expenditure (Table 3.1),[6, 17–19] equivalent in the UK to about eight times the amount spent on drugs (Fig. 3.1). This is not surprising given that about one-third of all patients with heart failure require admission to hospital each year,[16] and that hospital discharge rates for heart failure have been progressively rising over the last two decades.[7, 20] In the UK, the annual number of hospital admissions for heart failure now exceeds that for acute myocardial

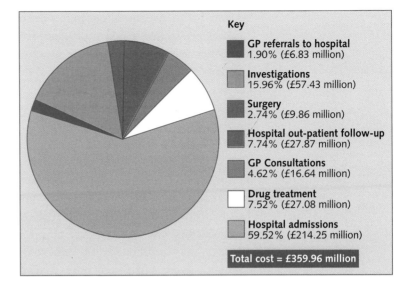

Key

GP referrals to hospital
1.90% (£6.83 million)

Investigations
15.96% (£57.43 million)

Surgery
2.74% (£9.86 million)

Hospital out-patient follow-up
7.74% (£27.87 million)

GP Consultations
4.62% (£16.64 million)

Drug treatment
7.52% (£27.08 million)

Hospital admissions
59.52% (£214.25 million)

Total cost = £359.96 million

FIG. 3.1 Components of spending on heart failure by the UK National Health Service between 1990 and 1991. (Redrawn from McMurray et al., 1993.)[18]

infarction.[7, 8] In the USA, heart failure is the commonest reason for hospitalization in people over the age of 65.[20] Health care utilization and the overall costs of care are greater in patients with more severe heart failure, primarily due to the need for more frequent hospitalization.[5]

Ideally, limited health care resources should be used to try and achieve maximum benefit for minimum expenditure, bearing in mind that the principal goals in the treatment of patients with any chronic illness should be to reduce symptoms and prolong survival. One of the most obvious conclusions is that treatment strategies which reduce the frequency or duration of hospitalization are likely to result in significant cost savings while simultaneously reducing associated patient morbidity. The ability of ACE inhibitors to reduce morbidity, and the costs associated with it, probably make them one of the most cost-effective therapies in modern medicine.

> Treatment strategies which reduce the frequency or duration of hospitalization are likely to result in significant cost savings while simultaneously reducing morbidity

Several large placebo-controlled studies have shown that ACE inhibitors can reduce the rate of hospitalization in patients with all severities of established heart failure as well as in individuals at risk of developing heart failure. ACE inhibitors also reduce the incidence of heart failure and the rate of related hospitalizations in

29

patients with asymptomatic left ventricular dysfunction. In the SOLVD prevention trial, more than 4000 asymptomatic patients with left ventricular ejection fractions less than 35% were randomized to receive either enalapril or placebo. Patients receiving enalapril were about 30% less likely to develop heart failure and about 30% less likely to require hospitalization than patients receiving placebo over a mean follow-up period of just over 3 years.[21]

These benefits suggest that the increasing utilization of ACE inhibitors may help diminish the economic burden of heart failure via a reduction in the frequency (and perhaps duration) of hospitalization. Several formal cost-effectiveness analyses have predicted that the cost of ACE inhibitor therapy in patients with heart failure would be at least offset by a reduced requirement for medical care, with net cost savings predicted in certain scenarios.[18, 19, 22] This is perhaps not surprising given that the cost of 1 year of treatment with an ACE inhibitor is equivalent to the cost of between one and two hospital bed-days.

> Increasing utilization of ACE inhibitors may help diminish the economic burden of heart failure via a reduction in frequency (and perhaps duration) of hospitalization

Despite accumulating evidence that treatment of heart failure with an ACE inhibitor probably represents one of the most cost-effective health care interventions in contemporary medicine (Table 3.2), it has been estimated that only about 30% of patients in the UK who stand to benefit from ACE inhibition are actually receiving it.[23, 24]

However, certain concerns still remain. As the various economic analyses have been based on clinical trials of relatively short duration, it has been suggested that ACE inhibitors may not reduce health care costs, but just postpone their impact. It has also been suggested that patients with heart failure may live longer and develop other illnesses, with additional cost implications. It is unlikely, however, that these potential 'catch-up' costs would manifest themselves to any significant extent given that ACE inhibitors extend life by only a relatively short period. Furthermore, patients with heart failure very rarely die a non-cardiac death.

TABLE 3.2 In the study of men born in 1913, the principal inclusion criterion was dyspnoea on exertion. A scoring system was used to try to separate cardiac from pulmonary causes. On the bases of their score, men were designated as having a particular stage of heart failure.

Cardiac disease scores

Previous myocardial infarction
Angina pectoris
Swollen legs at the end of the day
Nocturnal dyspnoea
Rales
Atrial fibrillation
Receiving treatment with diuretics and/or loop diuretics

Stage of heart failure	Criteria
Stage 0	No dyspnoea, no cardiac scores, no treatment
Stage 1	Cardiac scores but no dyspnoea or treatment
Stage 2	Cardiac scores and dyspnoea or cardiac scores and treatment
Stage 3	Cardiac scores and dyspnoea and treatment
Stage 4	Died from heart failure during follow-up

Manifest heart failure was considered present for those in stages 2, 3 or 4. Latent or possible heart failure was considered present for those in stage 1.

Conclusions

Heart failure is an increasingly common public health problem which, because of its considerable morbidity and dismal prognosis, imposes a massive socioeconomic burden on society. The devastating impact of heart failure on quality of life means that sufferers place major demands on health care systems, in particular because of their need for prolonged and recurrent hospitalization.

ACE inhibitors are an impressively cost-effective treatment because they can improve symptoms, delay disease progression and reduce mortality. Their earlier and more widespread use may help prevent the evolution of heart failure into an even more prevalent and costly epidemic. Further efforts must also be made to improve our understanding of the causes and pathophysiological basis of heart failure. New and more effective drug treatments are undoubtedly required and, perhaps most importantly, greater efforts must be made to institute risk factor interventions in individuals identified as being at risk of developing heart failure.

Greater efforts must be made to institute risk factor interventions in individuals identified as being at risk of developing heart failure

TABLE 3.3 In the National Health and Nutrition Examination Survey (NHANES), heart failure was considered to be present when a score of ≥3 was achieved using the following clinical scoring system.

Clinical variable	Score
Dyspnoea or difficulty breathing	
Trouble with breathing (shortness of breath)	1
Hurrying on the level or up a slight hill	1
Do you stop for breath when walking at your own pace?	2
Do you stop for breath after 100 m on the level?	2
Physical examination	
Heart rate (beats/min)	
91–110	1
≥111	2
Rales/crackles	
Either lower lung field	1
Either lower and either upper lung field	2
Jugulovenous distension	
Alone	1
Plus oedema	2
Plus hepatomegaly	2
Chest X-ray film	
Cephalization of pulmonary vessels	1
Interstitial oedema	2
Alveolar fluid plus pleural fluid	3
Interstitial oedema plus pleural fluid	3

TABLE 3.4 Predisposing factors to the development of heart failure in the Framingham study and five large clinical trials of vasodilator therapy in heart failures.

Aetiology	Framingham	V-HeFT I	CON-SENSUS	SOLVD (T)	V-HeFT II	SOLVD (P)
Ischaemic heart disease	30–45%	44%	73%	71%	53%	83%
Hypertension	77%	41%	21%	42%	48%	37%
Idiopathic	15%	N/A	15%	18%	N/A	9%
Diabetes	N/A	21%	22%	26%	20%	15%
Alcohol	N/A	40%	N/A	N/A	35%	N/A
Valvular	2%	5%	23%	N/A	N/A	N/A

V-HeFT, Vasodilator-Heart Failure Trial; CONSENSUS, Cooperative North Scandinavian Enalapril Survival Study; SOLVD, Studies of Left Ventricular Dysfunction; 'T' refers to SOLVD treatment trial; 'P' refers to SOLVD prevention trial.
N/A, Not applicable.

TABLE 3.5 Incidence of sudden cardiac death versus death from progressive pump failure in some of the large clinical trials of vasodilator therapy in heart failure.

	Sudden cardiac death	Progressive pump failure
V-HeFT I	45%[+]	
CONSENSUS	22% (P), 32% (E)	69% (P), 50% (E)[*]
SOLVD (T)	22% (P), 23% (E)	49% (P), 46% (E)
V-HeFT II	41% (H-ISDN), 31% (E)[**]	26% (H-ISDN), 38% (E)
SOLVD (P)	31% (P), 31% (E)	32% (P), 27% (E)

V-HeFT, Vasodilator-Heart Failure Trial; CONSENSUS, Cooperative North Scandinavian Enalapril Survival Study; SOLVD, Studies of Left Ventricular Dysfunction; 'T' refers to SOLVD treatment trial; 'P' refers to SOLVD prevention trial.
P, Placebo-treated patients; E, enalapril-treated patients; H-ISDN, hydralazine-isosorbide dinitrate-treated patients.
[+] Sudden death mortality in entire study population
[*] P = 0.001 placebo versus enalapril; [**] P = 0.015 hydralazine-isosorbide dinitrate versus enalapril.

TABLE 3.6 The annual cost of heart failure in the USA, France, the UK and the Netherlands. (From McMurray & Davie, 1996.)[25]

Countryon	Annual spending on heart failure	Percentage of total health care expenditure	Percentage of heart failure expenditure attributable to hospitalization
USA	$69 billion	1.5	71
France	FF11.4 million	1.9	64
UK	£360 million	1.2	60
Netherlands	NLG444 million	1.0	67

FF, French francs; NLG, Netherland guilders.

TABLE 3.7 Comparative costs of various medical interventions per quality adjusted life year (QALY). (From McMurray & Davie, 1996.)[25]

Intervention	Cost per QALY (£)
ACE inhibitor for mild to moderate heart failure	502
Pacemaker implant	1100
Valve replacement for aortic stenosis	1140
Hip replacement	1180
CABG for main stem stenosis with severe angina	2090
Renal transplantation	4710
Breast cancer screening	5780
Cardiac transplantation	7840
CABG for single-vessel disease with moderate angina	18 830
Renal haemodialysis in hospital	21 970

ACE, Angiotensin-converting enzyme; CABG, coronary artery bypass grafting.
*Cost calculated assuming 40% of patients are admitted to hospital for 1 day to start treatment while the remaining 60% start treatment in the community.

References

1 Sytkowski PA, Kannel WB, D'Agostino RB. Changes in risk factors and the decline in mortality from cardiovascular disease. *N Engl J Med* 1990; **322:** 1635–1641.
2 Department of Health. *The Health of the Nation.* HMSO, London, 1992.
3 Bonneux L, Barendregt J, Meeter K *et al.* Estimating clinical morbidity due to ischemic heart disease and congestive heart failure: the future risk of heart failure. *Am J Public Health* 1994; **84:** 20–28.

4 Stewart AL, Greenfield S, Hays RD *et al.* Functional status and well-being of patients with chronic conditions. *JAMA* 1989; **262:** 907–913.

5 Eriksson H, Svärdsudd K, Larsson B *et al.* Quality of life in early heart failure: the study of men born in 1913. *Scand J Prim Health Care* 1988; **6:** 161–167.

6 O'Connell JB, Bristow MR. Economic impact of heart failure in the United States: time for a different approach. *J Heart Lung Transplant* 1993; **13:** S107–S112.

7 McMurray J, McDonagh T, Morrison CE, Dargie HJ. Trends in hospitalization for heart failure in Scotland 1980–1990. *Eur Heart J* 1993; **14:** 1158–1162.

8 Parameshwar J, Poole-Wilson PA, Sutton GC. Heart failure in a district general hospital. *J R Coll Phys Lond* 1992; **26:** 139–142.

9 Kannel WB. Epidemiological aspects of heart failure. *Cardiol Clin* 1989; **7:** 1–9.

10 McKee PA, Castelli WP, McNamara PM, Kannel WB. The natural history of congestive heart failure: the Framingham study. *N Engl J Med* 1971; **285:** 1441–1446.

11 Ho KKL, Pinsky JL, Kannel WB, Levy D. The epidemiology of heart failure: the Framingham study. *J Am Coll Cardiol* 1993; 22 (suppl A): 6–13.

12 Ho KKL, Anderson KM, Kannel WB *et al.* Survival after the onset of congestive heart failure in Framingham heart study subjects. *Circulation* 1993; **88:** 107–115.

13 Schocken DD, Arrieta MI, Leaverton PE, Ross EA. Prevalence and mortality rate of congestive heart failure in the United States. *J Am Coll Cardiol* 1992; **20:** 301–306.

14 Franciosa JA. Why patients with heart failure die: hemodynamic and functional determinants of survival. *Circulation* 1987: 75 (suppl IV): 20–27.

15 The CONSENSUS Trial Study Group. Effects of enalapril on mortality in severe congestive heart failure. Results of the Cooperative North Scandinavian enalapril survival study. *N Engl J Med* 1987; **316:** 1429–1435.

16 The SOLVD Investigators. Effect of enalapril on survival in patients with reduced left ventricular ejection fractions and congestive heart failure. *N Engl J Med* 1991; **325:** 293–302.

17 Launois R, Launois B, Reboul-Marty J *et al.* Les coûtes de la séverité de la maladie: le case de l'insuffisance-cardiaque. *J Econ Med* 1990: 8: 395–412.

18 McMurray J, Hart W, Rhodes G. An evaluation of the cost of heart failure to the National Health Service in the UK. *Br J Med Econ* 1993; **6:** 99–110.

19 van Hout BA, Wielink G, Bousel HJ, Rutten FFH. Effects of ACE inhibitors on heart failure in the Netherlands: a pharmacoeconomic model. *Pharmacoeconomics* 1993; **3:** 387–397.

20 Ghali JK, Cooper R, Ford E. Trends in hospitalization rates for heart failure in the United States, 1973–1986. *Arch Intern Med* 1990; **150:** 769–773.

21 The SOLVD Investigators. Effect of enalapril on mortality and the development of heart failure in asymptomatic patients with reduced left ventricular ejection fractions. *N Engl J Med* 1992; **327:** 685–691.

22 Paul SD, Kuntz KM, Eagle KA *et al.* Costs and effectiveness of angiotensin converting enzyme inhibition in patients with congestive heart failure. *Arch Intern Med* 1994; **154:** 1143–1149.

23 Wheeldon NM, MacDonald TM, Flucker CJ, McKendrick AD, McDevitt DG, Struthers AD. Echocardiography in chronic heart failure in the community. *Q J Med* 1993; **86:** 17–23.

24 Clarke KW, Gray D, Hampton JR. Evidence of inadequate investigation and treatment of patients with heart failure. *Br Heart J* 1994; **71:** 584–587.

25 McMurray J, Davie A. The pharmacoeconomics of ACE inhibitors in chronic heart faillure. *Pharmacoeconomics* 1996; **9:** 188–197.

Pathophysiology of Heart Failure

SUMMARY POINTS

- Heart failure is a progressive disease: its natural history is variable, and there are often acute exacerbations
- Approximately 50% of patients are thought to die suddenly from ventricular tachycardia or fibrillation
- The progression of the disease may be explained by several mechanisms which result in a spiral of worsening heart failure, although not all patients progress to severe disease
- Loss of cardiac function can be divided into pump failure and myocardial failure
- Pump failure is due to abnormalities in the rhythm, valves or pericardium
- Myocardial failure results from myocyte loss, incoordinate contraction or extracellular and cellular remodelling
- The body's responses to heart failure include changes in the peripheral circulation, kidney, skeletal muscle, neurohumoral and sympathetic systems

Heart failure is a clinical syndrome caused by an abnormality of the heart and recognized by a characteristic pattern of haemodynamic, renal, neural and hormonal responses.[1] The two issues central to understanding the pathophysiology of heart failure are the nature of the abnormality of the heart and the characteristics of the body's response to that initiating cause. In chronic heart failure, the body's response determines the symptoms and signs.

Origins and dynamic nature of heart failure

It has been argued that the syndrome of heart failure is the response of the body to the heart's inability to maintain adequate blood pressure over a protracted period. Reflex, renal and hormonal responses to acute conditions such as hypovolaemia, haemorrhage and exercise are similar, if not identical, to the responses to heart failure. Thus, the sequelae of coronary heart disease in middle-aged or elderly patients in the last decade of the 20th century elicit a body response developed by evolution for an entirely different purpose.

Chronic heart failure should be regarded as a dynamic rather than a steady-state condition, as the function of the heart and its interaction with the circulation vary during the natural history and progression of the disease. Many patients with chronic heart failure develop acute exacerbations which are not always due to identifiable causes. The common clinical entity in which patients spontaneously improve and relapse with chronic heart failure has been termed undulating heart failure.

> Chronic heart failure should be regarded as a dynamic rather than a steady-state condition

Predictors of prognosis

Many clinical features have been shown to have prognostic significance in patients with heart failure, including:
* symptoms;
* exercise capacity;[2-5]
* signs;
* haemodynamics (left ventricular end-diastolic pressure);
* ventricular end-diastolic volume (on chest X-ray, echocardiography or as ejection fraction);[3]
* plasma hormone concentrations (noradrenaline, renin activity and atrial natriuretic peptide (ANP)).

ANP may be a particularly useful predictor of early heart failure.

However, such predictors often show only that patients who already have the features of heart failure will have a less favourable prognosis than asymptomatic individuals. The presence of heart failure predicts worsening heart failure, and worsening heart failure predicts death. Only a broad estimate of the prognosis in an individual patient is provided and there is poor discrimination in terms of prognosis among patients already classified as being in severe heart failure.

In severe heart failure, the best predictors of prognosis are:
* ejection fraction (a surrogate of end-diastolic volume);
* maximum oxygen consumption (a surrogate of maximum ventricular function);

• plasma sodium (a surrogate of renal and metabolic derangement).[4]

The two most powerful prognostic indicators in mild heart failure are the ejection fraction (end-diastolic ventricular volume) at rest and the peak oxygen consumption on exercise. The ejection fraction at rest is a surrogate for the extent of myocardial damage and the end-diastolic volume, rather than ventricular function. The peak oxygen consumption is an imprecise measure of cardiac reserve and ventricular function. An exercise test may be terminated by factors other than the limitations of the cardiovascular system, but the level of exercise achieved is a measure of the minimal capabilities of the cardiovascular system under stress.

> The two most powerful prognostic indicators in mild heart failure are the ejection fraction (end-diastolic ventricular volume) at rest and the peak oxygen consumption on exercise

Sudden death and arrhythmias

The mode of death in heart failure has been extensively studied, but firm conclusions are elusive. A substantial proportion of patients (up to 50%) are said to die suddenly, mostly from ventricular tachycardia/fibrillation, although asystole is a common terminal event in severe heart failure.[6–8] The remainder die from progression of heart disease. Sudden death due to an opportunistic arrhythmia cannot easily be distinguished from an expected arrhythmia in the context of an ischaemic event or progression of heart failure.

Sudden death has been defined as death within 6 h of the patient being known to be alive and well. Even if that time were reduced to a few minutes, there is still sufficient time for the onset of ischaemia to precede death, thus leading to an incorrect classification. A more useful, but still flawed, definition of sudden death is death from circulatory failure within 1 h of the onset of symptoms in a patient with advanced left ventricular dysfunction, whose heart failure symptoms have remained stable or improved over the previous 2–4 weeks, and in whom no other cause for circulatory collapse can be identified clinically.[7]

Arrhythmias (ventricular ectopics and non-sustained ventricular tachycardia) are common in patients with heart disease. Treatment with antiarrhythmic drugs is being evaluated in current trials, but at present this class of drug (with the possible exception of amiodarone) is not advantageous and may be harmful.

Arrhythmias are indicators of the severity of heart disease and not a powerful independent determinant of prognosis.

> Arrhythmias are indicators of the severity of heart disease and not a powerful independent determinant of prognosis

Spirals of heart failure

It has been demonstrated in animal models that the progression of ventricular dysfunction after myocardial infarction[9] or in response to hypertension can be altered by vasodilators. This suggests that the increased systemic vascular resistance in heart failure imposes an increased stress on the already damaged myocardium; this causes further damage to the heart muscle, followed by worsening heart failure, activation of neuroendocrine systems and a further increase of the systemic vascular resistance. The sequence is a spiral of heart failure with positive feedback (Fig. 4.1). However, evidence for this hypothesis is controversial.

Several other explanations have been put forward for the progression of heart failure (Fig. 4.1). One involves the retention of sodium and water secondary to hormonal activation and the haemodynamic effects on the kidney which follow the onset of ventricular dysfunction. Another is the biological process of remodelling (Fig. 4.2 and Table 4.1). This should not be confused with the change in heart size known to follow reduction of the circulating volume. Remodelling is a biological process involving the survival and orientation of cells in the myocardium. It may be

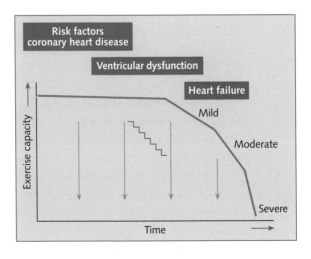

FIG. 4.1 Progression of heart failure.

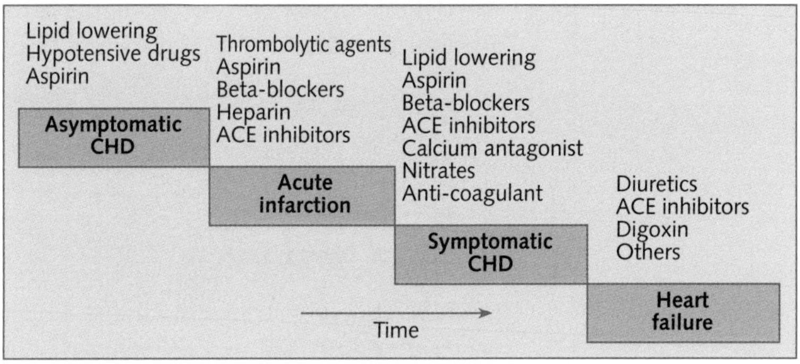

Lipid lowering Hypotensive drugs Aspirin	Thrombolytic agents Aspirin Beta-blockers Heparin ACE inhibitors	Lipid lowering Aspirin Beta-blockers ACE inhibitors Calcium antagonist Nitrates Anti-coagulant		
Asymptomatic CHD				
	Acute infarction			
		Symptomatic CHD	Diuretics ACE inhibitors Digoxin Others	
			Heart failure	

Time →

FIG. **4.2** Drugs and time in the treatment of coronary heart disease (CHD). ACE = Angiotensin-converting enzyme.

influenced by the renin–angiotensin system and growth factors within the myocardium, although the detailed pathophysiology is not understood.[10] Some authors believe that alteration of remodelling is a major mechanism of action of the benefit from treatment of heart failure with angiotensin-converting enzyme (ACE) inhibitors.[11]

TABLE 4.1 Shape changes in the heart after infarction 'remodelling'.	
Immediate	Dyskinesia of diseased myocardium Bulging of diseased myocardium Incoordinate contraction Necrosis and cell lengthening
Early (days to weeks)	Expansion of the infarcted myocardium Inflammation, scar formation, hypertrophy
Late (months to years)	Shape change of whole heart Enlargement of whole heart Fibrosis and hypertrophy

Several other vicious spirals are present in heart failure (Fig. 4.1). The muscle hypothesis[12] stresses the importance of:

- cytokine activation;
- skeletal muscle atrophy;
- signals from ergoreceptors in muscle.

The progression of atheroma in the coronary arteries and the occurrence of coronary events will obviously worsen heart failure and provide a new approach to treatment — prevention of reinfarction.

The final mechanism relates to activation of cytokines such as tissue necrosis factor-α (TNF-α) and interleukins, and the increased production of oxygen radicals. These damage cells in the myocardium and in skeletal muscle and may be particularly important in terminal heart failure, accounting for cardiac cachexia. Cell death may result from apoptosis (the programmed death of a cell by a non-inflammatory process).

Not all patients with heart failure progress to more severe disease (Fig. 4.3). Some die suddenly of an arrhythmia, but others will progress because of repeated episodes of myocardial ischaemia or the episodic destruction of myocytes. The appropriate and logical treatment depends critically on the presumed mechanism of progression, but as yet there is no means of predicting that in an individual patient.

> The appropriate and logical treatment depends critically on the presumed mechanism of progression

Reducing mortality

Diuretics prevent death in heart failure by reducing excessive sodium and water retention.[13–15] Nitrates and ACE inhibitors also reduce mortality,[11, 16–20] but they have no antiarrhythmic activity

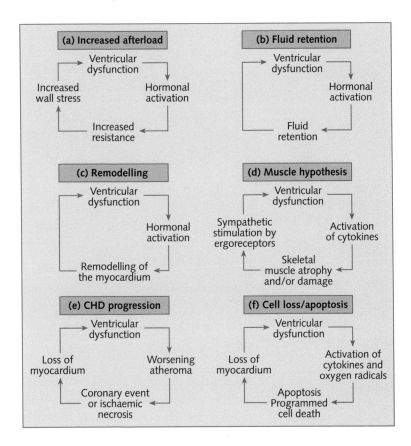

FIG. 4.3 Spirals of heart failure. CHD = Coronary heart disease.

and the mechanism of action remains unknown (Table 4.2). They may influence the frequency and occurrence of coronary events, but no direct effect on the myocardium has been shown.

TABLE 4.2 Putative mechanisms of action of angiotensin-converting enzyme (ACE) inhibitors.	
Vasodilation	Reduction of myocardial stress
Renal interaction with diuretics	Increased net loss of sodium
Remodelling	Ventricle shape Myocardial hypertrophy Fibrosis
Reduces ischaemic episodes	
Mechanism unrelated to ACE inhibition	

A popular hypothesis for the mechanism of angiotensin converting enzyme (ACE) inhibitors is that the reduction of afterload on the heart reduces the progression of damage to the myocardium. Alternatively, ACE inhibitors may increase renal blood flow and improve sodium homeostasis, thereby reducing the extent and occurrence of sodium overload. Clinical benefit in terms of exercise capacity could be accounted for if the improved sodium homeostasis resulted in reduced resistance in vascular beds and increase of blood flow to skeletal muscle on exercise.

> ACE inhibitors may increase renal blood flow and improve sodium homeostasis, thereby reducing the extent and occurrence of sodium overload

Another possible explanation is that ACE inhibitors directly and favourably affect the biological processes in the myocardium concerned with remodelling. They may thereby limit hypertrophy, prevent the deposition of collagen, prevent reinfarction and delay myocyte cell necrosis.

> ACE inhibitors may limit hypertrophy, prevent the deposition of collagen, prevent reinfarction and delay myocyte cell necrosis

Clinical causes of heart failure

Myocardial disease is by far the commonest cause of heart failure, and the commonest cause of myocardial failure is coronary heart disease (see Chapter 2). Heart failure develops in 50% of people who sustain a myocardial infarction.

Diastolic heart failure

The majority of patients attending hospitals for heart failure have abnormal systolic contraction, but systolic heart failure should be distinguished from diastolic heart failure, as they have different implications for treatment.[21, 22] In patients with diastolic heart failure, the stroke volume would be greater if filling during diastole had been more complete. In some conditions, such as hypertrophic obstructive cardiomyopathy, following valve replacement for aortic stenosis, hypertensive heart disease with hypertrophy, and angina pectoris, relaxation may be incomplete at end-diastole. The abnormality may be particularly evident if tachycardia is present.

Diastolic heart failure should be suspected in patients with symptoms of heart failure, hearts of a normal size and hypertrophy, myocardial ischaemia, or in the elderly. Even under these circumstances, a systolic abnormality may be present on exercise. In the presence of coronary heart disease, the key abnormality may not be incomplete relaxation of myocytes (affecting primarily isovolumic relaxation and rapid filling during early diastole), but rather incoordinate relaxation of different regions of the ventricle (affecting the later passive phase of ventricular filling). The evidence that diastolic function is a major factor limiting the maximal function of dilated hearts to pump blood is not compelling.

Patients with diastolic heart failure, particularly those with small hearts and angina or breathlessness as limiting symptoms in the presence of myocardial ischaemia or hypertrophy, may benefit from nitrates, vasodilator drugs or β-blockers. Such treatment results in reduced ischaemia in the endocardium, increased compliance and enhanced diastolic filling.

> Patients with diastolic heart failure may benefit from nitrates, vasodilator drugs or β-blockers

Acute heart failure

Acute heart failure, like the chronic disease, has many causes. The most common is myocardial ischaemia. The heart is critically dependent on a continuous supply of oxygen from the coronary circulation. Occlusion of a coronary artery causes contraction of heart muscle to cease within 60 s. Contractility is rapidly restored following the establishment of normal coronary flow, but some reduction of contractile function can persist for minutes, hours and even days after periods of ischaemia as short as 10 min. This condition has been called the stunned heart.[23, 24] Cell death occurs if the ischaemic period exceeds 15 min. If multiple episodes of transient ischaemia occur continually, normal function of the heart will never return. The term hibernating heart[25, 26] refers to a long-term reduction of contractility associated with continuing low blood flow and is similar to the older concept of chronic ischaemia.

> Contractility is rapidly restored following the establishment of normal flow, but some reduction of contractile function can persist for minutes, hours and even days

Chronic heart failure

The mechanisms responsible for the reduced contractility of heart muscle in chronic heart failure are more complex (Fig. 4.4; and see Chapter 2). Identification of a large heart with a low ejection fraction and minimal movement in systole does not necessarily mean that myocardial contractility is abnormal. Cardiovascular reflexes maintain the cardiac output at approximately 5 l/min. To achieve that in a large left ventricle, the ejection fraction and the movement of the ventricular wall must be reduced. A reduced ejection fraction in the presence of a large ventricle is a mathematical certainty and does not necessarily indicate diminished exercise capacity or cardiac reserve. There is a poor

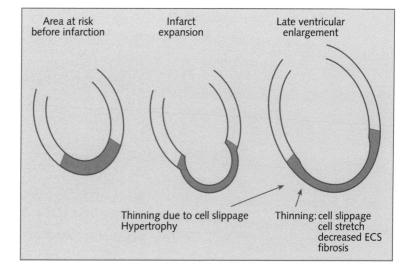

FIG. 4.4 Mechanisms responsible for the reduced contractility of heart muscle in chronic heart failure following myocardial infarction. ECS = Extracellular space.

> A reduced ejection fraction in the presence of a large ventricle is a certainty and does not necessarily indicate diminished exercise capacity or cardiac reserve

relation between the ejection fraction and the peak oxygen consumption on exercise.

A distinction should be made between pump failure, myocardial failure and inability of the myocyte to shorten.

Pump failure

Pump failure can be attributed to abnormalities of rhythm, valves or pericardium, whereas myocardial failure is due to pathology in cardiac muscle. The two most common abnormalities of the myocardium in coronary heart disease are loss of myocardial cells due to infarction, and incoordinate contraction. Any other loss of function must be attributable to extracellular or cellular abnormalities.

Myocardial failure

Myocardial failure may be due to cellular abnormalities of the myocyte[27, 28] or extracellular factors (Table 4.3). The major extracellular cause of heart failure is a change in the architecture and constituents of the myocardium, including a change of shape of the ventricle from pear-shaped to spherical, slippage of cells with thinning of the ventricular wall, and altered orientation of cells in the layers of the myocardium so that the cells lie more tangential to the ventricular cavity.

The major change in the constituents of the myocardium is an increase in the collagen content.[29] The myocardium normally contains 5% collagen, but this can rise to 25% in some forms of heart failure. The collagen is present as tendons, weaves and struts which form an extracellular structure that holds the myocytes in place and provides tensile strength (Table 4.4). Proteins in the extracellular space participate in many biological processes (Table 4.5). Extracellular changes may cause myocardial failure in the absence of any abnormality of contraction of individual myocytes.

> Extracellular changes may cause myocardial failure in the absence of any abnormality of contraction of individual myocytes

TABLE 4.3 Underlying causes of chronic heart failure due to the myocardium.

Loss of muscle

Incoordinate contraction and abnormal timing of contraction

Extracellular
Fibrosis, altered extracellular architecture, shape and size of ventricle slippage of cells, fibre orientation

Cellular
Change of cell structure
    Hypertrophy
    ? Hyperplasia
    ? Addition of sarcomeres

Change of cell function — systolic and/or diastolic

Calcium release/and or uptake	Response of contractile proteins to calcium
Receptor down-regulation	Altered contractile proteins (isoforms)
Reduced cyclic adenosine monophosphate	Altered phosphorylation of contractile proteins
Sarcoplasmic reticulum dysfunction	? Energy-deficient state
Reduced number of ion channels or pumps	

Many of these factors combine to cause systolic or diastolic failure. Diastolic heart failure is common in the presence of hypertrophy, fibrosis or ischaemia.

Myocytes

Much research has been undertaken to identify abnormalities of myocytes in the myocardium of the failing heart. There are undoubted histological abnormalities of cell structure, particularly if an active disease process is present. Myocytolysis and vacuolation of myocytes can be observed, and more subtle changes occur in the internal structure. Hypertrophy is common, indeed usual. Cells are in general wider, but only slightly longer. Increased width is more common in conditions where there is pressure overload, whereas increased length is observed in dilated or volume-overloaded ventricles. These changes lead to a heavier heart and can contribute to a thicker myocardium. Energy deficiency has been proposed as a cause of contractile failure,[30] but the evidence is weak.

There are undoubted histological abnormalities of cell structure, particularly if an active disease process is present

TABLE 4.4 Purpose of the collagen structure in the myocardium.

Maintains alignment of myocytes and muscle bundles

Prevents overstretching of the myocardium

Supports intramural coronary arteries

Transmits force

Stores energy in systole which contributes to relaxation

Determines shape and architecture of the heart

? The memory of the cardiac structure

80% type I, 12% type III, 4% (normal) to 25% (disease) by structural volume. Reactive or reparative.

TABLE 4.5 Proteins in the extracellular space.

Cell motility
   Migration
   Differentiation
Wound healing
Hypertrophy
Angiogenesis

TABLE 4.6 Control of myocardial contraction.

Action potential	
Calcium influx	
Release of calcium from the sarcoplasmic reticulum	Upstream regulation, e.g. catecholamines
Calcium transient	
Calcium bound to troponin C	
Activation of the myofibrillar adenosine biphosphatase	Downstream regulation, e.g. length dependence
Contraction	

Specific abnormalities of the function of intracellular structures have been shown in myocytes from the failing heart. Any reduction of function is due to a change in calcium sensitivity or availability (Table 4.6).

Body responses to heart failure

There are only a limited number of ways in which the body can respond to ventricular dysfunction associated with heart failure

TABLE 4.7 Body responses to heart failure.

Heart	
Structure	Loss of cells, abnormal fibre orientation, change of size and shape, fibrosis, hypertrophy
Function	Systolic and/or diastolic dysfunction
Circulation	
Structure	? Anatomical abnormality
Function	Altered neuroendocrine response, e.g. sympathetic system and renin–angiotensin
	Increased resistance – functional abnormality
Skeletal muscle	
Structure	Atrophy
Function	Abnormal biochemistry
	Increased weakness and fatigability

TABLE 4.8 Hormonal mediators in heart failure.

Constrictors	Dilators	Growth factors
Noradrenaline	Atrial natriuretic peptide	Insulin
Renin/angiotensin II	Prostaglandin E_2	Tumour necrosis factor-α
Vasopressin	and metabolites	Growth hormone
NPY	EDRF	Angiotensin II
Endothelin	Dopamine	Catecholamines
	Calcitonin gene-related peptide	Nitric oxide
		Oxygen radicals
		Cytokines

(Table 4.7). The principal changes are in the heart itself, the peripheral circulation, the kidney, and skeletal muscle. Activation of the neurohumoral system, activation of cytokines, and increased generation of oxygen radicals[31] have received considerable emphasis in recent years (Table 4.8, Fig. 4.5).

Neurohormonal activation

The sympathetic system is activated in mild heart failure, as is the renin–angiotensin system, but to a lesser degree (Fig. 4.5). Plasma aldosterone, antidiuretic hormone (vasopressin), prostaglandins and ANP are all elevated in severe heart failure. Numerous new peptides have been identified, many of which have powerful effects on sodium and water homeostasis and on systemic vascular resistance, although their role in the pathophysiology of heart failure is not yet established.

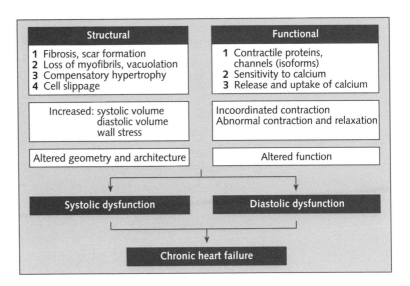

FIG. 4.5 Myocardial ischaemia.

ANP is released from the atria in response to stretch and causes both natriuresis and vasodilatation. In patients with heart failure, it is increased proportionally to the magnitude of both left and right atrial pressures. ANP may be a useful biochemical predictor of early heart failure.

The sensor that activates neurohumoral response remains conjectural, but baroreceptors in the heart and aorta, low-pressure sensors in the ventricles and atria, chemoreceptors in the carotid body and ergoreceptors in skeletal muscle may all be involved.

As diuretics are known to stimulate the renin–angiotensin system, part of the response to heart failure is in reality a response to treatment. The renin–angiotensin system is not activated in untreated patients with mild heart failure, whereas the sympathetic system and ANP are.[14,32,33] Increased plasma ANP and activation of the sympathetic system are the earliest neuroendocrine perturbations in heart failure.

> Increased plasma ANP and activation of the sympathetic system are the earliest neuroendocrine perturbations in heart failure

The sympathetic system

Plasma noradrenaline and adrenaline are elevated at rest in patients with heart failure.[34, 35] At similar but low levels of physical activity, the sympathetic system is more activated in heart failure than in normal individuals. At peak exercise, the opposite is true: plasma noradrenaline is higher in controls than heart failure patients. Sympathetic nerve signals are increased.[36] The sensitivity of most cardiovascular reflexes, including the baroreflexes, is blunted in heart failure. The myocardial content of noradrenaline is reduced in severe disease.

Studies on heart muscle obtained from patients with severe heart failure undergoing heart transplantation have shown that β-receptors are reduced in number. β-Blockers have been used to treat selected patients with heart failure. One possible mechanism of activity is that prevention of excessive sympathetic stimulation of the myocardium allows up-regulation of β-adrenergic receptors and a greater response of the myocardium to increased sympathetic stimulation on exercise. Alternative explanations are that tachycardia is avoided, that diastolic filling of the heart is improved, and that direct damage by catecholamines is diminished.

> β-Blockers have been used to treat selected patients with heart failure

Peripheral vascular resistance

Even when neurohormonal response is inhibited by drugs, systemic vacular resistance is still elevated at rest, and blood flow to skeletal muscle on exercise is markedly reduced.[37–40] Additional abnormalities also limit blood flow (Table 4.9). A popular but old hypothesis is that sodium is retained within smooth muscle, causing vasoconstriction. Alternative causes are endothelial cell swelling and abnormal endothelial cell function.[41] Until the putative abnormality is corrected, the resistance to blood flow during exercise in the skeletal muscle bed remains high and exercise performance is diminished. This mechanism probably explains why most inotropic drugs, vasodilators and ACE inhibitors do not increase exercise capacity when given acutely, but can do so (particularly the ACE inhibitors) after treatment has been continued for several weeks.[42]

Skeletal muscle

A recently emphasized and major response to heart failure is a change in the structure and function of skeletal muscle (Table 4.10).[43] In severe heart failure, cachexia is common, but muscle atrophy can occur even in moderate disease.[44–47] The cause of the

TABLE 4.9 Putative causes of increased peripheral resistance in chronic heart failure.

Reduced muscle mass

Anatomical
Thickened capillary basement membrane
Altered morphology of arteries and arterioles
Endothelial cell oedema
Microvascular infarction

Functional

Arterial vasoconstriction	Sodium–calcium exchange
	Neuroendocrine activation
	Unidentified peptide
	Reduced production or response to endothelin-derived relaxing factor or other endothelial cell products
Failure to dilate	Altered response to accumulated metabolites

TABLE 4.10 Skeletal muscle in heart failure.

Morphology

Quantity	Loss of muscle mass (or bulk)
Site	Localized to legs or general abnormality
	Orientation and fibre position
Quality	Atrophy, damage and/or necrosis
	Change of fibre type

Blood flow
ml/min reduced, ml/min per 100 ml variable

Metabolism
An inevitable consequence of atrophy and damage, or a specific change

Function
Weakness and/or increased fatigue

atrophy is unknown, but possible mechanisms are recurrent ischaemia on exercise, rest atrophy or a response to neurohormonal and cytokine activation. Atrophy of muscle may be more pronounced in the legs than arms and can be present in the diaphragm, contributing to shortness of breath. It may account for reported loss of strength,[48,49] increased fatigability[48] and metabolic abnormalities.[50] Because less muscle is present, blood flow to the lower limbs is reduced and vascular resistance increased. As peak oxygen consumption is related to muscle mass, there should be a relationship between achievable workload, peak oxygen consumption, muscle mass and total muscle blood flow.[49] Alterations in muscle efficiency would influence that relationship.

> A recently emphasized and major response to heart failure is a change in the structure and function of skeletal muscle

Activation of ergoreceptors from muscle may contribute to the sensation of fatigue and shortness of breath (Fig 4.6).[51] A further consideration is that a patient may not improve acutely on treatment because time is needed for recovery of the normal blood flow and function of skeletal muscle.[52]

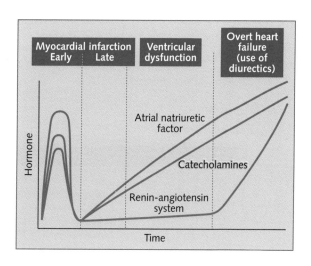

FIG. 4.6 Hormone activation in heart disease.

The kidney in heart failure

Clinical signs of heart failure (raised venous pressure, oedema) are largely due to the effect on the kidney (salt and water retention). In moderate heart failure, renal blood flow is reduced as a result of arterial vasoconstriction. Despite the fall of blood flow, the glomerular filtration rate is maintained as a result of greater constriction of the efferent arteries compared to the afferent arteries in the glomeruli. Filtration fraction is increased. In severe heart failure, renal blood flow is markedly reduced, glomerular filtration rate falls and the plasma urea and creatinine may increase. If the renin–angiotensin system is greatly activated by high-dose diuretics, the addition of ACE inhibitors can cause a further reduction of the glomerular filtration rate and an increase in plasma urea despite enhanced blood flow. This occurs because angiotensin II has a greater effect on the efferent artery than the afferent artery. A preferential reduction of resistance in the afferent artery leads to a fall in the pressures affecting the glomerular filtration rate.

> The clinical signs of heart failure (raised venous pressure, oedema) are largely due to the effect on the kidney (salt and water retention)

Causes of symptoms

The predominant symptoms of heart failure are breathlessness and fatigue (Table 4.11). Their origin is poorly understood.[43, 53, 54] In acute heart failure, shortness of breath is directly related to the left atrial pressure or the left ventricular end-diastolic pressure, but in patients with chronic disease treated with diuretics, the causes of breathlessness are less clear and almost certainly more complex. There is no simple correlation in this group of patients between peak oxygen consumption (a measure of exercise capacity) and estimates of left atrial pressure at peak exercise.

TABLE 4.11 Origin of symptoms on exercise in chronic heart failure.
Lungs
Increased stiffness due to raised venous pressure and lymphatic distension
Increased left atrial pressure
Increased physiological dead space
Increased respiratory rate
Weakness of diaphragm
Circulation
Reduced blood flow to skeletal muscle
Increased production of metabolites
Altered response to metabolites
Skeletal muscle
Rest atrophy
Ischaemic atrophy
Specific abnormality
Activation of ergoreceptors

Different types of exercise test give rise to different symptoms terminating exercise, despite the left atrial pressure at peak exercise being identical.[54] Changes in blood pH, plasma lactate, plasma potassium and other metabolic signals almost certainly contribute to shortness of breath in patients with chronic heart failure, in addition to changes in the lungs such as increased stiffness, increased ventilation and an increased physiological dead space.[51, 55–57]

The cause of fatigue is unknown. Patients with chronic heart failure have an increased resistance to blood flow in skeletal muscle at rest and on exercise. Metabolic signals may arise from the leg muscles due to stimulation of anaerobic metabolism (Fig. 4.7).[51] The mechanisms for shortness of breath and fatigue may both have their origins in skeletal muscle.

> The mechanisms for shortness of breath and fatigue may both have their origins in skeletal muscle

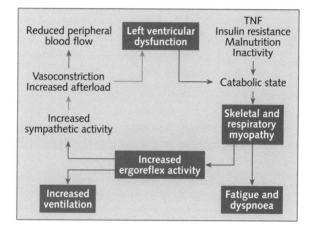

FIG. 4.7 Origin of symptoms: the muscle hypothesis. TNF = Tumour necrosis factor. From Coats *et al*.[12] with permission.

References

1 Poole-Wilson PA. Heart failure. *Med Int* 1985; **2**: 866–871.

2 Bittner V, Weiner DH, Yusuf S *et al*. Prediction of mortality and morbidity with a 6-minute walk test in patients with left ventricular dysfunction. *JAMA* 1993; **270**: 1702–1707.

3 Cohn JN, Johnson GR, Shabetai R *et al*. Ejection fraction, peak exercise oxygen consumption, cardiothoracic ratio, ventricular arrhythmias, and plasma norepinephrine as determinants of prognosis in heart failure. *Circulation* 1993; **87**: VI-5–VI-16.

4 Parameshwar J, Keegan J, Sparrow J, Sutton GC, Poole-Wilson PA. Predictors of prognosis in severe heart failure. *Am Heart J* 1992; **123**: 421–426.

5 Szlachic J, Massie BM, Kramer BL, Topic N, Tubau J. Correlates and prognostic implications of exercise capacity in chronic congestive heart failure. *Am J Cardiol* 1985; **55**: 1037–1042.

6 Francis GS. Development of arrhythmias in the patient with congestive heart failure: pathophysiology, prevalence and prognosis. *Am J Cardiol* 1986; **57**: 3B–7B.

7 Packer M. Sudden unexpected death in patients with congestive heart failure: a second frontier. *Circulation* 1985; **72**: 681–685.

8 Luu M, Stevenson WG, Stevenson LW, Baron K, Walden J. Diverse mechanisms of unexpected cardiac arrest in advanced heart failure. *Circulation* 1989; **80**: 1675–1680.

9 Pfeffer JM, Pfeffer MA, Braunwald E. Influence of chronic captopril therapy on the infarcted left ventricle of the rat. *Circ Res* 1985; **57**: 84–95.

10 Lindpainter K, Ganten D. The cardiac renin–angiotensin system. An appraisal of present experimental and clinical evidence. *Circ Res* 1991; **68**: 905–921.

11 Pfeffer MA, Braunwald, E, Moye LA. Effect of captopril on mortality and morbidity in patients with left ventricular dysfunction after myocardial infarction. *N Engl J Med* 1992; **327**: 669–677.

12 Coats AJS, Clark AL, Piepoli M, Volterrani M, Poole-Wilson PA. Symptoms and quality of life in heart failure: the muscle hypothesis. *Br Heart J* 1994; **72**: 36–39.

13 Slater JDH, Nabbaro JDN. Clinical experience with chlorothiazide. *Lancet* 1958; **1**: 124–126.

14 Bayliss J, Norell M, Canepa-Anson R, Sutton G, Poole-Wilson P. Untreated heart failure: clinical and neuroendocrine effects of introducing diuretics. *Br Heart J* 1987; **57**: 17–22.

15 Richardson A, Bayliss J, Scriven AJ, Parameshwar J, Poole-Wilson PA, Sutton GC. Double-blind comparison of captopril alone against frusemide plus amiloride in mild heart failure. *Lancet* 1987; **2**: 709–711.

16 The CONSENSUS Trial Study group. Effects of enalapril on mortality in severe congestive heart failure. Results of the Cooperative North Scandinavian enalapril survival study (CONSENSUS). The CONSENSUS trial study group. *N Engl J Med* 1987; **316**: 1429–1435.

17 Cohn JN, Johnson G, Ziesche S *et al.* A comparison of enalapril with hydralazine–isosorbide dinitrate in the treatment of chronic congestive heart failure. *N Engl J Med* 1991; **325**: 302–310.

18 Ball SG, Reynolds GW, Murray GD. ACE inhibitors after myocardial infarction. *Lancet* 1994; **343**: 1632.

19 The SOLVD Investigators. Effect of enalapril on survival in patients with reduced left ventricular ejection fractions and congestive heart failure. *N Engl J Med* 1991; **325**: 293–302.

20 Gruppo Italiano per lo Studio della Sopravvivenza nell'Infarto Miocardico. GISSI-3: effects of lisinopril and transdermal glyceryl trinitrate singly and together on 6-week mortality and ventricular function after acute myocardial infarction. *Lancet* 1994; **343**: 1115–1122.

21 Brutsaert DL, Sys SU. Relaxation and diastole of the heart. *Physiol Rev 1989*; **69**: 1228–1315.

22 Brutsaert DL, Sys SU, Gillebert TC. Diastolic failure: pathophysiology and therapeutic implications. *J Am Coll Cardiol* 1993; **22**: 318–325.

23 Bolli R. Mechanism of myocardial "stunning". *Circulation* 1990; **82**: 723–738.

24 Braunwald E, Kloner RA. The stunned myocardium: prolonged, postischemic ventricular dysfunction. *Circulation* 1982; **66**: 1146–1149.

25 Rahimtoola SH. A perspective on the three large multicenter randomized clinical trials of coronary bypass surgery for chronic stable angina. *Circulation* 1985; **72**: V123–V135.

26 Rahimtoola SH, Griffith GC. The hibernating myocardium. *Am Heart J* 1989; **117**: 211–221.

27 Jacob R, Gulch RW. Functional significance of ventricular dilation. Reconsideration of Linzbachis concept of chronic heart failure. *Basic Res Cardiol* 1988; **83**: 461–475.

28 Linzbach AJ. Heart failure from the point of view of quantitative anatomy. *Am J Cardiol* 1960; **5**: 370–380.

29 Weber KT, Brilla CC. Pathological hypertrophy and cardiac interstitium: fibrosis and renin-aldosterone system. *Circulation* 1991; **83**: 1849–1865.

30 Katz AM. Cardiomyopathy of overload. A major determinant of prognosis in congestive heart failure [see comments]. *N Engl J Med* 1990; **322**: 100–110.

31 Francis GS. Neurohumoral mechanisms involved in congestive heart failure. *Am J Cardiol* 1985; **55**: 15A–21A.

32 Francis GS, Benedict C, Johnstone DE *et al.* Comparison of neuroendocrine activation in patients with left ventricular dysfunction with and without congestive heart failure. *Circulation* 1990; **82**: 1724–1729.

33 Remes J, Tikkanen I, Fyhrquist F, Pyorala K. Neuroendocrine activity in untreated heart failure. *Br Heart J* 1991; **65**: 249–255.

34 Chidsey CA, Braunwald E, Morrow AG. Catecholamine excretion and cardiac stores of norepinephrine in congestive heart failure. *Am J Med* 1965; **39**: 442–451.

35 Chidsey CA, Harrison DC, Braunwald E. Augmentation of the plasma norepinephrine response to exercise in patients with congestive heart failure. *N Engl J Med* 1962; **267**: 650–654.

36 Leimbach WNJ, Wallin BG, Victor RG, Aylward PE, Sundlof G, Mark AL. Direct evidence from intraneural recordings for increased central sympathetic outflow in patients with heart failure. *Circulation* 1986; **73**: 913–919.

37 Zelis R, Flaim SF. Alterations in vasomotor tone in congestive heart failure. *Prog Cardiovasc Dis* 1982: **24**: 437–459.

38 LeJemtel TH, Maskin CS, Lucido D, Chadwick BJ. Failure to augment maximal limb blood flow in response to one-leg versus two-leg exercise in patients with severe heart failure. *Circulation* 1986; **74**: 245–251.

39 Wilson JR, Wiener DH, Fink LI, Ferraro N. Vasodilatory behaviour of skeletal muscle arterioles in patients with nonedematous chronic heart failure. *Circulation* 1986; **74**: 775–779.

40 Wilson JR, Ferraro N. Exercise intolerance in patients with chronic heart failure: role of impaired nutritive flow to skeletal muscle. *Circulation* 1984; **69**: 1079–1087.

41 Katz SD, Biasucci L, Sabba C *et al.* Impaired endothelium-mediated vasodilation in the peripheral vasculature of patients with congestive heart failure. *J Am Coll Cardiol* 1992; **19**: 918–925.

42 Lipkin DP, Poole-Wilson PA. Treatment of chronic heart failure: a review of recent trials. *Br Med J* 1985; **291**: 993–996.

43 Poole-Wilson PA, Buller NP, Lipkin DP. Regional blood flow, muscle strength and skeletal muscle histology in severe congestive heart failure. *Am J Cardiol* 1988; **62**: 49E–52E.

44 Dunnigan A, Staley NA, Smith SA *et al.* Cardiac and skeletal muscle abnormalities in cardiomyopathy: comparison of patients with ventricular tachycardia or congestive heart failure. *J Am Coll Cardiol* 1987; **10**: 608–618.

45 Drexler H, Hiroi M, Riede U, Banhardt U, Meinertz T, Just H. Skeletal muscle blood flow, metabolism and morphology in chronic congestive heart failure and effect of short- and long-term angiotensin-converting enzyme inhibition. *Am J Cardiol* 1988; **62**: 82E–85E.

46 Sullivan MJ, Green HJ, Cobb FR. Skeletal muscle biochemistry and histology in ambulatory patients with long-term heart failure. *Circulation* 1990; **81**: 518–527.

47 Lipkin DP, Jones DA, Round JM, Poole-Wilson PA. Abnormalities of skeletal muscle in patients with chronic heart failure [published errata appear in *Int J Cardiol* 1988; **19**. 396 and *Int J Cardiol* 1988; **20**: 161]. *Int J Cardiol* 1988; **18**: 187–195.

48 Buller NP, Jones D, Poole-Wilson PA. Direct measurement of skeletal muscle fatigue in patients with chronic heart failure. *Br Heart J* 1991; **65**: 20–24.

49 Volterrani M, Clark AL, Ludman PF *et al.* Predictors of exercise capacity in chronic heart failure. *Eur Heart J* 1994; **15**: 801–809.

50 Massie BM, Conway M, Rajagopalan B *et al.* Skeletal muscle metabolism during exercise under ischemic conditions in congestive heart failure. Evidence for abnormalities unrelated to blood flow. *Circulation* 1988; **78**: 320–326.

51 Clark A, Coats A. The mechanisms underlying the increased ventilatory response to exercise in chronic stable heart failure. *Eur Heart J* 1992; **13**: 1698–1708.

52 Sinoway LI, Minotti JR, Davis D *et al.* Delayed reversal of impaired vasodilation in congestive heart failure after heart transplantation. *Am J Cardiol* 1988; **61**: 1076–1079.

53 Lipkin DP, Poole-Wilson PA. Symptoms limiting exercise in chronic heart failure. *Br Med J* 1986; **292**: 1030–1031.

54 Lipkin DP, Canepa-Anson R, Stephens MR, Poole-Wilson PA. Factors determining symptoms in heart failure: comparison of fast and slow exercise tests. *Br Heart J* 1986; **55**: 439–445.

55 Sullivan MJ, Higginbotham MB, Cobb FR. Increased exercise ventilation in patients with chronic heart failure: intact ventilatory control despite hemodynamic and pulmonary abnormalities. *Circulation* 1988; **77**: 552–559.

56 Buller NB, Poole-Wilson PA. Mechanism of the increased ventilatory response to exercise in patients with chronic heart failure. *Br Heart J* 1990; **63**: 281–283.

57 Clark Al, Poole-Wilson PA, Coats AJS. The relationship between ventilation and carbon dioxide production in patients with chronic heart failure. *J Am Coll Cardiol* 1992: **20**: 1326–1332.

Symptoms and Signs of Heart Failure

SUMMARY POINTS

- The symptoms of heart failure are generally non-specific
- The signs of heart failure are generally insensitive
- Clinical scoring systems are interesting but of limited use
- The diagnosis of heart failure in general practice has been shown to be strewn with hazards
- Clinical evaluation must be combined with objective assessment

The reader may wonder why it is necessary to spend valuable time giving consideration to the symptoms and signs of heart failure, but heart failure is difficult to define, to measure and, particularly, to diagnose. Surely every general practitioner knows that the classical symptoms are dyspnoea, ankle oedema and fatigue, and is competent enough at clinical examination to confirm or refute a diagnosis once it is suggested by the patient's symptoms. The fact is, however, that no one symptom, sign or combination of symptoms and/or signs is absolutely sensitive or specific for the diagnosis of heart failure.

Of course, this is true of diagnostics in any field of medicine — the days when diagnosis was based solely on the intercourse between patient and doctor, on history and examination, without any investigations, have long since passed into medical history — but it is perhaps particularly true for the diagnosis of heart failure. The situation is further complicated by the difficulty of establishing a 'gold standard' test for the objective diagnosis of heart failure and even of establishing a consensus on the definition.

Heart failure is difficult to define, to measure and, particularly, to diagnose

Sensitivity and specificity

It is necessary to have an objective measure of whether heart failure is present or not in order to establish the sensitivity, specificity and positive and negative predictive value of any given symptom or sign. Sensitivity refers to the percentage of patients with heart failure correctly identified. Specificity refers to the percentage of patients without heart failure correctly identified. Positive predictive value refers to the percentage of patients with a given symptom or sign who actually have heart failure. Negative predictive value refers to the percentage of patients without a given symptom or sign who actually do not have heart failure.

Clearly, the ideal symptom or sign would have 100% sensitivity, specificity and positive and negative predictive value; however, as a degree of mutual exclusivity is implied, it is equally clear that in most cases sensitivity, specificity and positive and negative predictive values are all much nearer 50% (what they would be if a symptom or sign had no discriminatory value whatsoever). Clinically, the most useful parameters are sensitivity (which helps distinguish true positives from false negatives) and positive predictive value (which helps distinguish true positives from false positives).

> Sensitivity, specificity and positive and negative predictive value all help define the utility of a diagnostic feature in clinical practice

Studies showing difficulty in diagnosis

Several studies have assessed the usefulness of different symptoms or signs or combinations of symptoms and/or signs in the diagnosis of heart failure. However, the interpretation of their findings is influenced by a number of factors:
- the patient population (for example, selected inpatients versus unselected patients from general practice);
- prior treatment (for example, diuretics);
- time-course of the condition (acute and chronic heart failure have very different clinical profiles);
- nature of the objective measure chosen as the 'gold standard' against which to set symptoms and signs.

Of these, the last point is by far the most important.

Diagnosis based on symptoms

The classical symptoms of heart failure are dyspnoea, ankle oedema and fatigue. Dyspnoea on exertion is common in the general population and more so in the obese. It may be a symptom of respiratory disease and can be confused with angina of effort. It is hardly surprising, therefore, that it cannot be used as the sole criterion for the diagnosis of heart failure. Orthopnoea and paroxysmal nocturnal dyspnoea are less common in the general population than dyspnoea on exertion alone, and are therefore likely to be more specific, but less sensitive, for the diagnosis of heart failure. Ankle oedema is not always due to heart failure; in fact, it is not even mostly due to heart failure, so even if allowance is made for misinterpretation of fat ankles or a firm desire for slim ankles, it is hardly surprising that it is very variable in sensitivity and specificity, depending on the patient population. Little attention has been paid to the symptom of fatigue, not least because it is so widespread in the general population.

> The classical symptoms of heart failure are dyspnoea, ankle oedema and fatigue, but none of them is particularly useful

At least four studies have examined the sensitivity, specificity and positive and negative predictive value of symptoms for the diagnosis of heart failure.

The Duke group[1] gave sensitivity, specificity and positive predictive value for dyspnoea on exertion, orthopnoea, paroxysmal nocturnal dyspnoea and ankle oedema. Paroxysmal nocturnal dyspnoea was less sensitive and more specific than dyspnoea on exertion; orthopnoea was less sensitive and more specific than paroxysmal nocturnal dyspnoea, and ankle oedema was about the same as orthopnoea.

Chakko *et al.*[2] gave sensitivity, specificity and positive and negative predictive value for orthopnoea and ankle oedema with somewhat greater sensitivity and positive predictive value, but somewhat less specificity.

Stevenson and Perloff's data[3] can be interpreted as showing that orthopnoea had a sensitivity of 91% and a specificity of 100% and that ankle oedema had a sensitivity of 23% and a specificity of 100%.

The findings of Echeverria *et al.*[4] can be interpreted to give sensitivity, specificity, positive and negative predictive value for dyspnoea on exertion, orthopnoea, paroxysmal nocturnal dyspnoea and ankle oedema. The results are greater sensitivity and less specificity for dyspnoea on exertion, orthopnoea and paroxysmal nocturnal dyspnoea than the Duke group, and about the same for ankle oedema (Table 5.1). It is difficult for the general reader to draw any conclusion from these studies, except that none of these symptoms as studied is consistently useful.

		Harlan et al.[1]	Chakko et al.[2]	Stevenson and Perloff[3]	Echeverria et al.[4]
TABLE 5.1 Sensitivity, specificity, positive (PPV) and negative predictive value (NPV) of symptoms for the diagnosis of heart failure (%).					
Dyspnoea on exertion	Sensitivity	66			97
	Specificity	52			15
	PPV	23			63
	NPV				75
Orthopnoea	Sensitivity	21	66	91	73
	Specificity	81	47	100	40
	PPV	2	61	100	65
	NPV		37	64	50
Paroxysmal nocturnal dyspnoea	Sensitivity	33			50
	Specificity	76			45
	PPV	26			58
	NPV				38
Ankle oedema	Sensitivity	23	46	23	23
	Specificity	80	73	100	70
	PPV	22	79	100	54
	NPV		37	18	38

Diagnosis based on signs

The clinical signs of heart failure reflect the consequences more than the causes of heart failure. Thus, left ventricular dilatation is reflected in signs of cardiomegaly (displaced apex beat, increased area of cardiac dullness, third heart sound); fluid retention is reflected in signs of congestion (ankle oedema, jugular venous distension, pulmonary crackles); low cardiac output is reflected in signs of poor perfusion (decreased proportional pulse pressure); and neuroendocrine activation is reflected in signs of increased sympathetic tone (resting tachycardia).

The most useful signs are probably the most subtle: third heart sound, increased width of cardiac dullness and displaced apex beat

At least seven studies have examined the sensitivity, specificity and predictive value of signs for the diagnosis of heart failure (Table 5.2). The Duke group[1] gave sensitivity, specificity and positive predictive value for resting tachycardia, pulmonary crackles, ankle oedema, third heart sound and jugular venous distension. None was particularly sensitive, although all were fairly specific, and only third heart sound had substantial positive predictive value. Heckerling et al.[5] reported that increased width of cardiac dullness was very sensitive and quite specific. O'Neill et al.[6] reported that displacement of the apex beat was a bit more specific, but quite a lot less sensitive. Chakko et al.[2] gave sensitivity, specificity and positive and negative predictive value for pulmonary crackles, ankle oedema, third heart sound and jugular venous distension. They found greater sensitivity, but less specificity than the Duke group. Butman et al.[7] gave sensitivity, specificity and positive and negative predictive value for pulmonary crackles, third heart sound and jugular venous distension. In terms of sensitivity and specificity, their results were close to the Duke group, but positive predictive value was much higher.

Stevenson and Perloff's data[3] may be interpreted as giving a specificity and positive predictive value of 100% for pulmonary crackles, ankle oedema and jugular venous distension, and a high sensitivity for third heart sound. The findings of Echeverria et al.[4] can be interpreted to give sensitivity, specificity and positive and negative predictive value for pulmonary crackles, ankle oedema, third heart sound, jugular venous distension and displaced apex beat. Their results are much the same order of magnitude as those reported by Chakko et al.

It is difficult for the reader to draw any general conclusion from these studies, but they do imply that third heart sound and displaced apex beat are consistently useful, whereas pulmonary crackles, ankle oedema and jugular venous distension are probably not.

Diagnosis based on clinical scoring systems

A number of clinical scoring systems based on combinations of symptoms and/or signs (and/or non-specialist non-invasive tests such as electrocardiograms and chest X-rays) have been devised as an aid to diagnosis. These scores have shown variable correlation with objective criteria such as left ventricular ejection fraction as assessed by radionuclide ventriculography (Table 5.3). Marantz et al.[8]

TABLE 5.2 Sensitivity, specificity, positive (PPV) and negative predictive value (NPV) of signs for the diagnosis of heart failure.

	Harlan et al.[1]	Heckerling et al.[5]	O'Neill et al.[6]	Chakko et al.[2]	Butman et al.	Stevenson and Perloff[3]	Echeverria et al.[4]
Resting tachycardia							
Sensitivity	7						
Specificity	99						
PPV	6						
NPV							
Pulmonary crackles							
Sensitivity	13			66	24	19	70
Specificity	91			84	100	100	35
PPV	27			87	100	100	62
NPV				61	35	17	44
Ankle oedema							
Sensitivity	10			46		23	40
Specificity	93			73		100	70
PPV	3			79		100	67
NPV				46		18	44
Third heart sound							
Sensitivity	31			73	68	98	63
Specificity	95			42	73	14	55
PPV	61			66	86	88	68
NPV				85	48	50	50
Jugular venous distension							
Sensitivity	10			70	57	58	47
Specificity	97			79	93	100	65
PPV	2			85	95	100	67
NPV				62	47	28	45
Increased percussion distance							
Sensitivity			94				
Specificity			67				
PPV							
NPV							
Displaced apex beat							
Sensitivity			59				60
Specificity			76				50
PPV			59				64
NPV			77				45
Proportional pulse pressure							
Sensitivity						91	
Specificity						8	
PPV						91	
NPV						87	

TABLE 5.3 Sensitivity, specificity, positive (PPV) and negative predictive value (NPV) of clinical scoring systems for the diagnosis of heart failure.

	Sensitivity	Specificity	PPV	NPV
Marantz *et al.*[8]				
Framingham	63	63		
Duke	73	54		
Boston	50	78		
Carlson *et al.*[9]	90	85	73	95
Mattleman *et al.*[10]	86	88	84	89
Cease and Nicklas[11]	88	84	78	91
Eagle *et al.*[12]				
Physician	76	76	71	81
Score	79	80	76	83

correlated three different sets of clinical criteria (Framingham, Boston and Duke) with left ventricular ejection fraction. Only Framingham criteria were equally sensitive and specific. Duke criteria were more sensitive, but less specific, and Boston criteria were less sensitive, but more specific. Clearly, a diagnosis based on satisfaction of all three sets of criteria would be much less sensitive, but much more specific.

Carlson *et al.*[9] correlated their own (Boston) criteria with pulmonary capillary wedge pressure and found good sensitivity and specificity. Mattleman *et al.*[10] devised a score based on dyspnoea, pulmonary crackles, presence of Q waves on the electrocardiogram and radiological evidence of cardiomegaly to estimate ejection fraction with ~90% sensitivity, specificity and positive and negative predictive value. Cease and Nicklas[11] devised a score based on heart rate, pulse pressure, radiological heart size and radiological chest size to obtain an estimate of left ventricular ejection fraction with similar predictive values. Eagle *et al.*[12] devised a score based on radiological heart size, radiological evidence of pulmonary venous hypertension, blood pressure, history of hypertension, apex beat and third heart sound to get a measure of similar value (and, furthermore, made a comparison with cardiologists' estimates based on history, examination, electrocardiograph and chest X-ray).

Again, it is difficult for the general reader to draw any conclusion from these studies. This reflects the fact that clinical scoring systems are perhaps rather more useful in epidemiological studies than in clinical practice.

The most useful clinical scoring systems are those that combine symptoms and signs with the results of simple tests

Diagnosis of heart failure in general practice

Recent studies have evaluated the accuracy of diagnosis of heart failure in general practice in newly diagnosed patients, in diuretic-treated patients and in a mix of the two. In all reports, the positive predictive value of pre-existing diagnoses of heart failure as compared with more objective forms of assessment was low (64% compared with Boston criteria,[13] 55% compared with Boston criteria plus additional clinical criteria,[13] 41% compared with echocardiography[14] and 18% compared with open-access echocardiography.[15]) Women were more commonly misdiagnosed than men, and obese individuals were more commonly misdiagnosed than the non-obese.

Overall, heart failure due to left ventricular systolic dysfunction is at least as likely to be underdiagnosed as overdiagnosed in general practice, at least partly due to the poor sensitivity and specificity of the symptoms and signs. However rigorous with respect to assessment of symptoms, signs and even clinical scoring systems, diagnosis of heart failure in general practice is likely to remain haphazard, and will continue to require objective substantiation. It is really not possible to propose a reliable framework for the diagnosis of heart failure: whatever criteria or combination of criteria are chosen, the incidence of false positives and false negatives is so high as to require objective assessment in almost all cases.

Studies confirm that the diagnosis of heart failure in general practice is at best difficult and at worst frequently erroneous

So how can heart failure be diagnosed?

Although a clinical diagnosis of heart failure secondary to left ventricular systolic dysfunction can be difficult, it is possible to identify patients who are likely to have heart failure on clinical grounds alone, although the diagnosis must be supported by objective measurement of left ventricular function. Take for example a number of patients complaining of dyspnoea and fatigue:

1   Patient A is a middle-aged to elderly man who is not excessively overweight and who has a past history of myocardial infarction. He complains of dyspnoea on exertion, but not orthopnoea or paroxysmal nocturnal dyspnoea; he may or may not have ankle swelling. Examination reveals normal pulse and blood pressure, slight jugular venous distension, displaced apex beat, clear lungs and slight ankle swelling. The probability of heart failure must be high. Objective assessment is required to guide further treatment, even if it is not required for initial diagnosis.

2   Patient B is a middle-aged woman who is obese but has no past history of note. She complains of dyspnoea on exertion, orthopnoea, occasional paroxysmal nocturnal dyspnoea and frequent ankle swelling. Examination reveals normal pulse and blood pressure; the jugular venous pulse is invisible; the apex beat is impalpable; the heart sounds are almost inaudible; the chest is clear and the ankles are slightly swollen. This patient is much less likely to have heart failure. Objective assessment may be required to reassure both patient and physician that no further treatment is required.

3   Patient C is an elderly woman who seems increasingly run-down. She has a murmur, but little past history of note. The patient complains of dyspnoea on exertion, but not orthopnoea, paroxysmal nocturnal dyspnoea or ankle swelling. Examination reveals resting tachycardia, decreased proportional pulse pressure, jugular venous distension, displaced apex beat, heart sounds obscured by a murmur, clear lungs and slightly swollen ankles. She may very well have heart failure secondary to left ventricular systolic dysfunction, but is at least as likely to have critical valvular disease. Objective assessment is required to resolve the very real uncertainty which surrounds her case.

4   Patient D is a middle-aged man who is obese and smokes heavily. He complains of dyspnoea on exertion, but no orthopnoea, paroxysmal nocturnal dyspnoea or ankle swelling. Examination reveals normal pulse and blood pressure; the jugular venous pulse is invisible; the apex beat is impalpable; the heart sounds are almost inaudible; the chest is wheezy and the ankles are not swollen. He may have heart failure but is more likely to have angina of effort or developing chronic lung disease. Objective assessment of left ventricular systolic function may be required after exclusion of these other possibilities (also, if necessary, by objective means).

Past history is an integral part of the clinical assessment. Subjective assessment must be combined with objective assessment to ensure that treatment is appropriate

As a general rule, besides the clinical assessment of symptoms and signs of heart failure, it is necessary wherever possible to make an objective assessment of left ventricular systolic function before making a firm diagnosis of heart failure. This avoids false-positive diagnosis with the risk of unnecessary, incorrect or even potentially hazardous treatment. It also helps avoid false-negative diagnosis with the risk of omission of proven effective treatment. In addition, it is important to remember that heart failure is not always due to irreversible impairment of left ventricular systolic function; some cases, such as pericardial or valvular disease, are readily amenable to corrective treatment, for example by surgery. Objective assessment ensures that treatment is always appropriate.

Conclusion

The diagnosis of acute left ventricular failure is easy, but the diagnosis of chronic heart failure secondary to left ventricular systolic dysfunction is a very different matter. Symptoms and signs are not enough to identify such patients; instead, it is important to remember the background of the patient and that heart failure is a syndrome, not a diagnosis. Always ask: 'if this patient does have heart failure, why does he have heart failure and why is he presenting with it now?' Sometimes these questions will be impossible to address, but the epidemiology of heart failure tells us that they are easily answered in the vast majority of cases and provide the key to diagnosis.

It is easy to show that no single symptom or sign is adequately sensitive or specific for the diagnosis of heart failure. It can also be shown that combinations of symptoms and/or signs may be more specific, but are less sensitive and therefore have less positive predictive value. Scoring systems which incorporate symptoms and signs as well as the results of simple non-invasive non-specialist investigations may come closer to day-to-day clinical practice, but objective assessment shows that they are not accurate enough to pin individual clinical fates on (although they may be good enough to use as epidemiological tools). Optimal evaluation and, more importantly, optimal treatment of the patient depend on both objective assessment and clinical evaluation.

Diagnosis of heart failure secondary to left ventricular systolic
dysfunction is difficult. Only objective assessment is good enough

References

1 Harlan WR, Oberman A, Grimm R, Rosati RA. Chronic congestive heart
failure in coronary artery disease: clinical criteria. *Ann Intern Med* 1977; **86:**
133–138.

2 Chakko S, Woska D, Martinez H *et al.* Clinical, radiographic, and
hemodynamic correlations in chronic congestive heart failure: conflicting
results may lead to inappropriate care. *Am J Med* 1991; **90:** 353–359.

3 Stevenson LW, Perloff JK. The limited reliability of physical signs for estimating
hemodynamics in chronic heart failure. *JAMA* 1989; **261:** 884–888.

4 Echeverria HH, Bilsker MS, Myerburg RJ, Kessler KM. Congestive heart
failure: echocardiographic insights. *Am J Med* 1983; **75:** 750–755.

5 Heckerling PS, Wiener SL, Moses VK, Claudio J, Kushner MS, Hand R.
Accuracy of precordial percussion in detecting cardiomegaly. *Am J Cardiol*
1991; **91:** 328–334.

6 O'Neill TW, Barry M, Smith M, Graham IM. Diagnostic value of the apex beat.
Lancet 1989; **1:** 410–411.

7 Butman SM, Ewy GA, Standen JR, Kern KB, Hahn E. Bedside cardiovascular
examination in patients with severe chronic heart failure: importance of rest or
inducible jugular venous distension. *J Am Coll Cardiol* 1993; **22:** 968–974.

8 Marantz PR, Tobin JN, Wassertheil-Smoller S *et al.* The relationship between
left ventricular systolic function and congestive heart failure diagnosed by
clinical criteria. *Circulation* 1988; **77:** 607–612.

9 Carlson KJ, Lee DC-S, Goroll AH, Leahy M, Johnson RA. An analysis of
physicians' reasons for prescribing long-term digitalis therapy in outpatients. *J
Chron Dis* 1985; **38:** 733–739.

10 Mattleman SJ, Hakki A-H, Iskandrian AS, Segal BL, Kane SA. Reliability of
bedside evaluation in determining left ventricular function: correlation with left
ventricular ejection fraction determined by radionuclide ventriculography. *J Am
Coll Cardiol* 1983; **1:** 417–420.

11 Cease KB, Nicklas JM. Prediction of left ventricular ejection fraction using
simple quantitative clinical information. *Am J Med* 1986; **81:** 429–436.

12 Eagle KA, Quetermous T, Singer DE *et al.* Left ventricular ejection fraction:
physician estimates compared with gated blood pool scan measurements. *Arch
Intern Med* 1988; **148:** 882–885.

13 Remes J, Miettinen H, Reunanen A, Pyorala K. Validity of clinical diagnosis of
heart failure in primary health care. *Eur Heart J* 1991; **12:** 315–321.

14 Wheeldon NM, MacDonald TM, Flucker CJ, McKendrick AD, McDevitt DG,
Struthers AD. Echocardiography in chronic heart failure in the community. *Q
J Med* 1993; **86:** 17–23.

15 Francis CM, Caruana L, Kearney P *et al.* Open access echocardiography in
management of heart failure in the community. *Br Med J* 1995; **310:** 634–636.

Investigating the Patient with Heart Failure

SUMMARY POINTS

- Initial assessment should include both a detailed history and a physical examination
- Renal function must be confirmed before the administration of nephrotoxic drugs such as diuretics and angiotensin-converting enzyme inhibitors
- One of the principal investigations is an electrocardiogram which can provide information about ventricular damage, left ventricular hypertrophy, myocarditis or dilated cardiomyopathy
- A posteroanterior direct chest radiograph can reveal the presence of dilation, elevated pressure in the pulmonary vessels or pleural effusions
- Echocardiography is a non-invasive technique which can provide information about cardiac structure and function without the use of ionizing radiation
- The aetiological basis of the disease may be elucidated by the use of radionucleotide ventriculography, exercise testing, radionuclide myocardial profusion scanning, coronary angiography analytical entrychiology, and 24-h ambulatory electrocardiogram monitoring

It is important for all doctors who see patients with suspected heart failure to ensure that an accurate and complete diagnosis is reached. Failure to do so may mean not only that the patient is denied appropriate treatment, but also that misdiagnosed patients may go untreated or receive unnecessary and potentially harmful treatment. A sure diagnosis of heart failure cannot be made unless there is some objective evidence of cardiac dysfunction in the presence of symptoms. Even then, the nature, extent and aetiology of the condition should be established with as much certainty as is appropriate to the clinical setting. Any coexisting diseases which may provoke or aggravate it, or which may affect subsequent management, must be taken into account.

A sure diagnosis of heart failure cannot be made unless there is some objective evidence of cardiac dysfunction in the presence of symptoms

Results of investigations should be interpreted in the context of the whole clinical picture. Even if a patient is shown to have impaired left ventricular systolic function, it is not necessarily the cause of his or her current symptoms. The investigating doctor must keep an open mind at all times.

The size of the problem of chronic heart failure within the community means that for most patients the general practitioner (GP) will be responsible for orchestrating and acting upon the initial basic investigations. This will be done in conjunction with outpatient cardiology services which, rightly, are becoming more available to GPs on an open-access basis. Every GP should have a clear plan of investigation for the patient with suspected heart failure. The question of who should be referred to specialist cardiology departments for further assessment is addressed below.

For most patients, the GP will be responsible for orchestrating and acting upon the initial basic investigations

Clinical assessment

Investigation of the patient with suspected heart failure begins with careful clinical assessment. Although symptoms may be the only indicator as to the diagnosis during the initial consultation, there are no accepted clinical diagnostic criteria for heart failure. Even if there were, physicians would often disagree about the presence or absence of symptoms and signs in any one patient, limiting their clinical usefulness.[1] Scoring systems based on symptoms, signs and, in some instances, chest radiographs appear to have a sensitivity and specificity of only about 60–70% at best for diagnosing left ventricular systolic dysfunction when compared to radionuclide ventriculograms.[2–4]

Having said that, a full history and physical examination may reveal important aetiological factors for heart disease, such as previous myocardial infarction or heavy alcohol intake. It may also reveal an obvious alternative cause for the patient's symptoms, or evidence of coexisting disease. The cardinal symptoms of exertional dyspnoea, fatigue and ankle oedema are common and may be caused by several non-cardiac diseases. Furthermore, patients at risk of ischaemic heart disease and subsequent left ventricular damage form a substantial part of the population at risk from other disorders, such as chronic obstructive pulmonary disease and renal impairment.

Most of the time-honoured signs of heart failure, such as peripheral oedema, pulmonary rales and elevated jugular venous pressure are brought about by renal retention of salt and water and have a firm relationship with central haemodynamics in acute,[5] but not chronic, heart failure. Chronic heart failure is characterized by the activation of several compensatory mechanisms which alter the physical signs, often leading to the absence of peripheral oedema and pulmonary rales.[6]

Treatment with diuretics may remove all signs of the condition. The exception to this is the third heart sound which is considered to be a reliable sign of heart failure with an elevated ventricular filling pressure, if present.[7] It can however be overlooked and physicians again differ on its presence in any one patient.[8] If signs of congestion are found at the initial consultation, a diuretic may need to be started pending further investigation.

> Treatment with diuretics may remove all signs of the condition, with the exception of the third heart·sound

Thus, physical examination may be entirely normal in chronic heart failure even though objective evidence of major systolic dysfunction is found on subsequent investigation.[9] On the other hand, up to 40% of people diagnosed clinically as having heart failure have normal systolic function.[10, 11] This group includes individuals with other non-cardiac causes for their signs and symptoms. Some, particularly the elderly, will have presumed diastolic dysfunction. This condition, characterized by abnormal diastolic filling of the left ventricle, is difficult to diagnose confidently by non-invasive means, particularly in an older patient.[12] It may, however, produce exercise intolerance and dyspnoea similar to that found in isolated left ventricular systolic dysfunction. Such patients are important to recognize because they have nothing to gain from angiotensin-converting enzyme (ACE) inhibitor treatment.

> Physical examination may be entirely normal in chronic heart failure even though objective evidence of major systolic dysfunction is found on subsequent investigation

As a clinical diagnosis of heart failure is unreliable, further investigations are required even if the doctor is convinced of the cause of the patient's symptoms and signs. Attaching the label of chronic heart failure to a patient should be regarded as only the starting point in the diagnostic process.

> Attaching the label of chronic heart failure to a patient should be regarded as only the starting point in the diagnostic process

Basic investigations

Every patient with suspected heart failure should undergo certain basic investigations (Table 6.1). It is to be hoped that GPs will have access to them all, but the availability of echocardiography varies from area to area. Once that is done, it should be apparent whether or not the patient has appreciable cardiac dysfunction. Further investigation may then be indicated to learn more about the aetiology of the condition or to determine whether intervention is required. At this point, the patient should be referred to a cardiology clinic.

> Every patient with suspected heart failure should undergo certain basic investigations

TABLE 6.1 Basic investigations for patients with suspected heart failure.
Blood tests
Full blood count
Urea and electrolytes
Thyroid function tests
Urinalysis
Electrocardiogram
Chest X-ray
Echocardiogram

Blood tests

These are readily available to all GPs and are relatively inexpensive.

Full blood count

Full blood count may reveal the presence of anaemia which may provoke or aggravate heart failure. Polycythaemia may suggest the presence of severe respiratory disease with a degree of ventilatory failure.

Urea, creatinine and electrolytes

Renal disease may not only mimic heart failure with signs and symptoms of fluid retention, but may also affect its treatment, which is dependent on functioning kidneys. Baseline renal function should be measured and documented prior to the administration of potentially nephrotoxic drugs, such as diuretics and ACE inhibitors. Following the initiation of ACE inhibitors, renal function and electrolytes should be measured at regular intervals.

> Renal disease may not only mimic heart failure with signs and symptoms of fluid retention, but may also affect its treatment

ACE inhibition may lead to a medical autonephrectomy in patients with unilateral renal artery stenosis. Unfortunately, this can occur without appreciable deterioration in urea and creatinine. Such renal vascular disease is not uncommon in the population with coronary artery disease, particularly those with a history of peripheral vascular disease. If it is suspected, specialist assessment either by renal angiography or by an isotope study will be required prior to the administration of ACE inhibitors.

Electrolyte disturbance is unusual in untreated heart failure but common among patients taking diuretics, who frequently exhibit hypokalaemia. Hyponatraemia makes the initiation of ACE inhibitors more hazardous as the patient is likely to have a very active renin–angiotensin–aldosterone system. Early referral to a cardiology clinic is recommended.

Thyroid function tests

Thyroid dysfunction (both hypo- and hyperthyroidism) may aggravate or provoke heart failure. Hyperthyroidism may first present with atrial fibrillation, particularly in elderly patients.

Urinalysis

This simple and inexpensive technique can be performed in the surgery with instant results. Proteinuria and/or haematuria may indicate the presence of renal disease such as glomerulonephritis or the nephrotic syndrome which may cause fluid retention and so mimic the signs of heart failure.

> Proteinuria and/or haematuria may indicate the presence of renal disease causing fluid retention and so mimicking the signs of heart failure

Electrocardiography

The ECG is, as it has been for many years, a principal investigation in patients with suspected or known heart disease. Every GP has access to electrocardiography either in the surgery or at the local hospital. It is simple and quick to perform, inexpensive, non-invasive and most doctors are able to interpret the results.

A normal ECG is rare in the context of chronic heart failure;[11] however, an abnormal ECG does not necessarily mean that heart failure is the cause of any symptoms or signs.

> An abnormal ECG does not necessarily mean that heart failure is the cause of any symptoms or signs

Several pieces of information pertaining to possible causes of heart failure can be obtained from an ECG:

Evidence of ventricular damage or disease

Infarction

In western countries, the commonest cause of heart failure is left ventricular systolic dysfunction secondary to loss of functioning myocardium from ischaemic necrosis. Previous infarction may show on the ECG by:

1 The presence of pathological Q waves (>40 ms in duration or with a depth > 25% of the height of the ensuing R wave) in leads I, II aVF, or V2–V6 (Fig. 6.1).

2 Low-amplitude QRS complexes in the standard limb leads and loss of R-wave amplitude in the anterior leads indicating loss of left ventricular myocardial mass. Generally small complexes in all the leads may suggest the presence of a pericardial effusion or hypothyroidism.

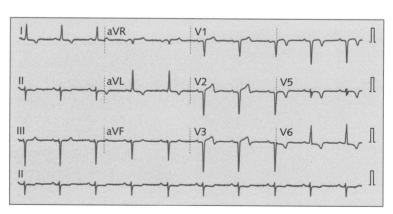

FIG. 6.1 Twelve lead ECG — anterior Q wave MI.

3   Left bundle branch block (Fig. 6.2). If due to infarction, this usually indicates substantial damage to the interventricular septum as the left bundle branch is a relatively diffuse structure within the septum. It may however occur due to other pathology. In contrast, right bundle branch block may be a normal occurrence in people without heart disease.

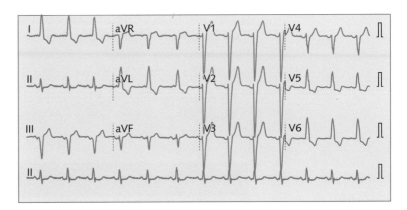

FIG. 6.2 Twelve lead ECG — left bundle branch block.

The ECG may be relatively normal even in the context of substantial damage from previous infarction. Between 10% and 20% of pathological Q waves regress substantially over time and a further 50% regress partially.[12] Q waves may not appear at all where there is an area of intramural infarction (even a large one) with a shell of epicardium surviving.[13] On the whole, there is a poor correlation between QRS findings and measured left ventricular function.[12]

> On the whole, there is a poor correlation between QRS findings and measured left ventricular function

Left ventricular hypertrophy (LVH)

This most commonly arises from long-standing hypertension, but may also indicate the presence of aortic stenosis or hypertrophic cardiomyopathy. LVH is of prognostic importance in itself, as it leads to a substantial increase in mortality.[14] Compared to echocardiography, ECG is a relatively insensitive test for LVH.[15]

> Compared to echocardiography, ECG is a relatively insensitive test for LVH

LVH is *suggested* by increased QRS voltages in those leads which reflect the electrical activity of the left ventricle (so-called voltage criteria; Table 6.2). Additionally, there may be ST-T repolarization abnormalities with down-sloping ST-segment depression and asymmetrical T-wave inversion, particularly in the lateral chest leads (so-called LV strain pattern (Fig. 6.3)). The presence of an LV strain pattern makes the voltage criteria more specific for LVH. In its absence, isolated voltage criteria for LVH must be interpreted in terms of the body habitus of the individual. In young, healthy, thin-chested individuals the ECG will frequently exceed QRS voltage criteria for LVH.

> In young, healthy, thin-chested individuals the ECG will frequently exceed QRS voltage criteria for LVH

TABLE 6.2 Electrocardiogram features suggestive of left ventricular hypertrophy.

• Net positivity in I + net negativity III	>1.7 mV
• R in aVL	>1.2 mV
• S in V1 + R in V5	>3.5 mV
• Greatest R + deepest S	>4.0 mV

Myocarditis/dilated cardiomyopathy

The ECG is usually abnormal with a variety of non-specific findings, including bundle branch blocks, non-specific interventricular conduction defects and asymmetrically inverted T waves in most of the standard limb leads.

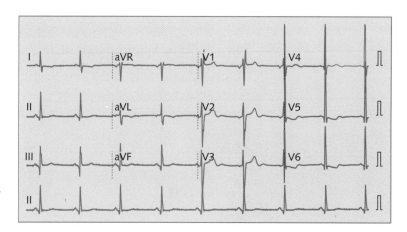

FIG. 6.3 Twelve lead ECG — left ventricular hypertrophy with 'strain pattern' and an inferior MI.

Presence of brady- or tachyarrhythmias

Atrial fibrillation (AF) and atrial flutter (considered here as one condition) are two of the commonest arrhythmias encountered in general practice and may accompany any cardiac condition which causes heart failure. AF with a fast ventricular rate may by itself precipitate heart failure, but even when the ventricular rate is controlled, its onset may cause a deterioration in the patient with reduced systolic function. Loss of atrial systole may cause a reduction of some 20% in cardiac output. In addition AF may lead to the formation of intracardiac thrombus with the danger of embolic events, particularly stroke. The risk of thromboembolism is increased in the presence of other cardiac disease, such as reduced left ventricular function. Thus, diagnosing AF is important as consideration should be given to anticoagulating the patient with warfarin and possible cardioversion to sinus rhythm.

> Diagnosing AF is important as consideration should be given to anticoagulating the patient with warfarin and possible cardioversion to sinus rhythm

Similarly, bradycardia may precipitate or worsen existing heart failure. Priority should be given to stopping any negatively chronotropic drugs, but even then a pacemaker may be required to improve the cardiac output.

Patients with chronic ischaemic left ventricular dysfunction have a higher than normal frequency of ventricular ectopic beats. There is a correlation between the frequency of ectopic beats and the severity of the left ventricular dysfunction, and their presence is an independent risk factor for sudden death. In the post myocardial infarct patient, suppression of ectopic beats by antiarrhythmic drugs has not been proven to improve the prognosis, and may worsen it.[16]

> In the post myocardial infarct patient, suppression of ectopic beats by antiarrhythmic drugs has not been proven to improve the prognosis, and may worsen it

More serious arrhythmias, such as paroxysmal ventricular tachyarrhythmias, are unlikely to be captured on a single resting ECG and usually require one or more 24-h Holter monitor ECGs to be detected.

Chest radiography

Although chest radiography has become less important since the advent of echocardiography, it remains worthwhile. Every GP has access to radiographic services, usually with an accompanying radiology opinion.

A standard posteroanterior (PA) erect chest radiograph is required in the patient with suspected heart failure. Certain features should be examined closely.

Cardiac silhouette

The heart size is recorded from a chest X-ray as the ratio of its transverse diameter to the internal diameter of the thorax (the chest–thorax ratio or CTR). In normal individuals, the CTR is <0.5. However, this is a crude parameter; the heart may appear enlarged on chest X-ray due to left or right ventricular dilatation, or left or right ventricular hypertrophy (Fig. 6.4).[17] It is usually not possible to distinguish between these conditions by examining the external cardiac contours.

Furthermore, as the left ventricle is not significantly dilated in many patients with left ventricular impairment, the CTR may well be normal. Heart size may also be normal in the presence of significant hypertrophy, as the hypertrophied wall often encroaches on the ventricular cavity and the heart size may not increase until ventricular failure with dilatation occurs. Thus, cardiomegaly on a

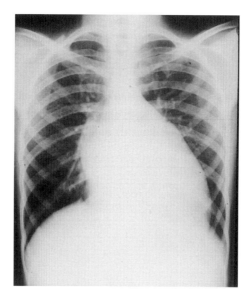

FIG. 6.4 Chest X-ray — cardiomegaly.

chest X-ray alone is neither a sensitive nor a specific means of detecting left ventricular systolic dysfunction.[18]

Cardiomegaly on a chest X-ray alone is neither a sensitive nor a specific means of detecting left ventricular systolic dysfunction

Left atrial enlargement may more easily be distinguished by a double contour adjacent to the right heart border. Such a finding is usually due to rheumatic mitral valve disease.

A grossly enlarged cardiac shadow, with loss of contours, should alert the doctor to the possibility of a chronic pericardial effusion and prompt urgent echocardiography. A similar cardiac shadow is sometimes found in dilated cardiomyopathy. In cases of acute effusion, the chest X-ray is usually normal, even when significant cardiac tamponade is present, as the pericardium does not have an opportunity to expand.

Although visualization of calcium within a valve on X-ray suggests valvular pathology, it is a common finding in elderly individuals with no valvular dysfunction. Pericardial calcification is found in 50% of patients with constrictive pericarditis but may be almost impossible to see on a standard PA film and is more easily detected on a lateral view.[17]

Lung fields and pulmonary vasculature

Left ventricular failure and mitral valve disease may both elevate left atrial pressure and consequently the pulmonary venous pressure. As this becomes more severe, progression of radiological findings is observed. Initially, blood flow is diverted to the upper zones of the lungs such that on an erect film the calibre of the upper zone vessels equals or exceeds lower-zone vessels at a similar distance from the hila. As this proceeds, fluid is exuded into the lung interstitium and causes normally invisible septa within the lung to become oedematous and visible on the film as Kerley A and B lines. At a more severe stage, alveolar oedema may occur with its characteristic bilateral and symmetrical perihilar distribution giving rise to a bat's-wing appearance with sparing of the peripheral lung fields, which may contain Kerley B lines.

As with pulmonary rales on auscultation, interstitial and alveolar oedema on a chest X-ray are more usual features of acute left heart failure (Fig. 6.5) and may be absent in many patients with chronic left ventricular impairment due to compensatory mechanisms.

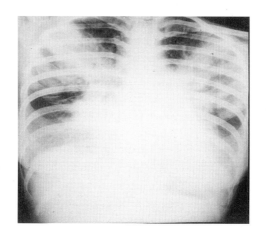

FIG. 6.5 Chest X-ray — acute heart failure with pulmonary oedema.

Pleural effusions may develop in left heart failure. They are usually bilateral, but if they are unilateral the right side is commonly affected.

The lung fields may, of course, show pulmonary pathology such as emphysematous changes or pulmonary fibrosis. These may be the cause of the patient's symptoms, even in the presence of heart failure. Pulmonary hypertension is not evident on chest X-ray until it is severe and revealed by enlargement of the pulmonary arteries with peripheral pruning. This is not usually seen in patients with raised pulmonary artery pressure due to left ventricular failure alone.

> Pulmonary pathology may be the cause of the patient's symptoms, even in the presence of heart failure

Echocardiography

Echocardiography is rapidly establishing itself as the primary investigation in patients with suspected heart failure. Most general hospitals now have at least one echo machine, and many GPs have direct access to echocardiography on an outpatient request basis. As this service is likely to expand, it is all the more important that doctors in primary care become familiar with the advantages and the limitations of echocardiography and understand its basic principles.

> It is important that doctors in primary care become familiar with the advantages and the limitations of echocardiography and understand its basic principles

The appeal of echocardiography lies in its ability to give information about cardiac structure and function completely non-invasively and without using ionizing radiation. An average scan takes about 20–30 min and provides information about the myocardium, endocardium (including the valves) and pericardium (Fig. 6.6).

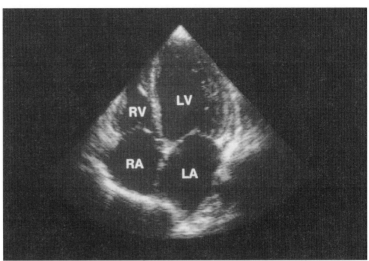

FIG. 6.6 Echocardiogram — apical four chamber view of a normal heart.

The amount of information obtained is dependent on the technical quality of the pictures which, in turn, depends on the operator finding clear echo windows on the chest wall (points at which the ultrasound beam may pass unimpeded). Not all the views may be obtained in any one patient, particularly if he or she is elderly, has chronic respiratory disease with a degree of hyperinflation, or is obese. Many patients with heart failure fall into at least one of these categories. However, the views of the left ventricle are usually adequate for assessment of systolic function.[19]

Echocardiography assesses the left side of the heart best, and is much less useful for looking at the right side. An irregular or rapid ventricular rhythm, such as occurs with atrial fibrillation or frequent ectopic beats, makes interpretation of the echocardiogram difficult, particularly with regard to left ventricular function and wall motion.

A full echocardiographic examination assesses most if not all of the following aspects of cardiac structure and function.

Left ventricular systolic function

The major question asked of echocardiography in suspected heart failure is whether left ventricular systolic function is impaired and, if so, how severe it is. A quantitative measurement of global left ventricular systolic function is obtained by calculating the left ventricular ejection fraction (LVEF). This is the stroke volume (the difference between the end-diastolic and end-systolic volumes) expressed as a percentage of the left ventricular end-diastolic volume. LVEF is a good marker of the severity of left ventricular systolic dysfunction as it has been correlated with survival and outcome in heart failure[20] and has been used as the measure of left ventricular function in many large trials.[21, 22] However, calculation of LVEF by echocardiography using a method such as the Simpson's biplane method is too time-consuming to perform accurately in the clinical setting and may be open to many errors. Hence, for the most part, it remains a research tool.

> Calculation of LVEF by echocardiography is too time-consuming to perform accurately in the clinical setting and may be open to many errors

In most clinical settings, global left ventricular systolic function is therefore assessed visually by an observer based on his or her experience of normal and abnormal function. This type of qualitative rather than quantitative assessment is usually sufficient and tends to be fairly reproducible, particularly when differentiating between good, moderate and poor function.[19] Differences between observers arise when finer scales of assessment are used.

Fractional shortening is a surrogate measurement of global left ventricular function. Quicker and easier to measure than the ejection fraction, it is based on the change in the internal diameter of the left ventricle as measured by M-mode echocardiography during the cardiac cycle. This measurement, taken at one level in the ventricle, does not necessarily account for the presence of discrete areas of infarction within the ventricle.

Wall motion

Areas of infarction can usually be seen on an echocardiogram as a region of the left ventricular myocardium which may be thinned and showing abnormal systolic contraction, or wall motion. Wall motion is assessed visually and as such is subjective, although fairly reproducible. An area of myocardium showing abnormal wall motion may be described as:
- hypokinetic: with reduced systolic contraction;

- akinetic: non-contractile;
- dyskinetic: the timing and/or direction of systolic motion differs from that expected and at one extreme may represent a ventricular aneurysm.

There is a correlation between the extent of such abnormal wall motion within a left ventricle and the ejection fraction.[23]

Cardiac dimensions: M-mode

M-mode cardiography was one of the first echocardiography techniques to be developed. It measures the diameter of the left ventricular cavity and the thickness of the wall at standard points. Thus, LVH may be identified and its severity quantified. Echocardiography is 5–10 times more sensitive than ECG in detecting the presence of LVH and will detect its presence in up to 30% of patients with hypertension (Fig. 6.7).[15]

> Echocardiography is 5–10 times more sensitive than ECG in detecting the presence of LVH

Left ventricular end-diastolic and end-systolic diameters may be measured to detect the presence of left ventricular dilatation, as may occur in left ventricular dysfunction. Left atrial size can also be measured and may be increased in mitral valve disease (including incompetence secondary to left ventricular dilatation and annular dilatation) and in the presence of atrial fibrillation alone.

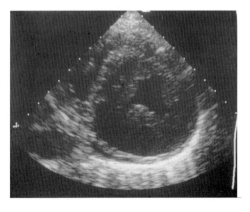

FIG. 6.7 Echocardiogram — short axis view of LV showing severe left ventricular hypertrophy.

Assessment of valves: Doppler and colour-flow Doppler

Echocardiography has revolutionized the assessment of valves and has reduced the need for invasive tests. Valves can be visually assessed using two-dimensional echocardiography for evidence of structural abnormalities such as:

- thickening of the cusps;
- cusp fusion;
- calcification;
- prolapse of a leaflet.

Colour-flow Doppler can be used to visualize the direction of blood flow through a valve and detect incompetence. In left ventricular dysfunction there is often mitral incompetence due to annular dilatation accompanying left ventricular dilatation (Plate 6.1, facing p. 84). Doppler echocardiography allows the velocity and timing of blood flow through valves to be measured and hence the gradient across the valve to be calculated, thus detecting valvular stenosis.

Doppler detection of at least a minor amount of tricuspid regurgitation in the majority of individuals allows for the calculation of the pulmonary artery systolic pressure and the identification of pulmonary hypertension. This may be elevated not only in left ventricular dysfunction and mitral valve disease but also in pulmonary and pulmonary vascular disease.

Other structural abnormalities

Echocardiography can also be used to detect a number of other structural abnormalities which may or may not cause symptoms and signs, and to assess their effects on the circulation. These include left-to-right shunts, as occur in atrial and ventricular septal defects. As little as 20–50 ml of pericardial fluid can be seen on an echo and it may be possible to detect features of cardiac tamponade. Clot visualized on the endocardial surface of a non-contractile segment within the left ventricle after a myocardial infarction is an indication for anticoagulation.

> Echocardiography can be used to detect a number of structural abnormalities which may or may not cause symptoms and signs

Additional investigations

The basic investigations described above should reveal the general nature of the cardiac problem; for example, whether or not the patient has left ventricular systolic dysfunction. For most purposes, an accurate ejection fraction will not be required, and echocardiography will be sufficient to exclude or confirm

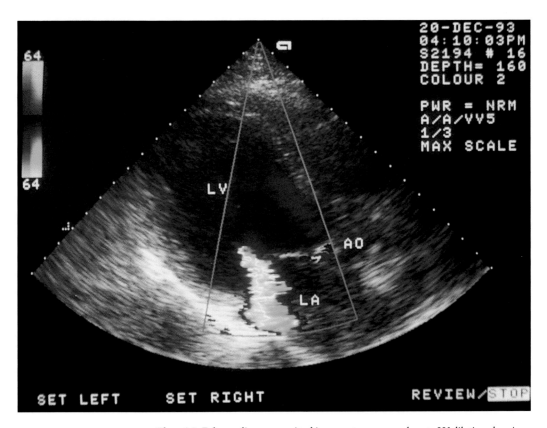

Plate 6.1 Echocardiogram—mitral incompetence secondary to LV dilation showing on colour flow doppler.

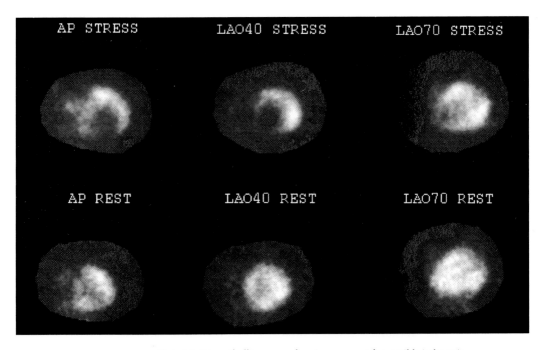

Plate 6.2 Stress thallium scan showing an area of reversible ischaemia.

ventricular systolic dysfunction. This, together with the additional information gained, makes it the preferred first-line investigation. There are instances, however, when it may be desirable or necessary to use radionuclide ventriculography, particularly when inadequate pictures are obtained by echocardiography or when there is debate as to whether a ventricle is mildly impaired or normal.

> Radionuclide ventriculography may be used when inadequate pictures are obtained by echocardiography or when there is debate as to whether a ventricle is mildly impaired or normal

Identifying the aetiology of the left ventricular dysfunction now becomes an issue. In most cases this will already have been revealed through findings such as a previous myocardial infarction or LVH on the ECG or echocardiogram. In others it may not be as clear and additional investigations may be required (Table 6.3).

TABLE 6.3 Additional investigations in patients with heart failure.

Radionuclide ventriculography
Assessment of myocardial perfusion/ischaemia
   Exercise testing
   Radionuclide myocardial perfusion scanning
   Coronary angiography
24-h ambulatory electrocardiogram monitoring

Radionuclide ventriculography

This form of cardiac imaging is good at quantifying ventricular systolic function by means of calculating the left ventricle ejection fraction; in that respect it is easier than echocardiography. The ejection fraction obtained by radionuclide ventriculography tends to be more reproducible than that obtained by echocardiography, because it is averaged over several hundred beats.

Radionuclide ventriculography yields relatively little information about cardiac structure other than obvious wall motion abnormalities and ventricular dilatation. In this respect it is very much inferior to echocardiography. As with echo, it is affected by an irregular ventricular rate, although computing software can ameliorate this to some extent. The technique is influenced to a greater degree by anterior wall function than by other areas of the heart and so an anterior infarction will affect the ejection fraction measured by radionuclide ventriculography more than an infarction in another site. As there is wide variation in the normal range quoted by different departments within the UK, any result should be interpreted with reference to the standard values of the department concerned.

> Radionuclide ventriculography yields relatively little information about cardiac structure other than obvious wall motion abnormalities and ventricular dilatation

The major drawback to radionuclide ventriculography is the need to administer doses of ionizing radiation. In addition, it is more expensive to perform on a scan-per-scan basis than echocardiography, and is less widely available. Few centres allow GPs to request the service directly.

Assessment of myocardial perfusion/ischaemia

There is good reason to look for evidence of coronary artery disease and reversible ischaemia in patients who have left ventricular dysfunction at rest. It has been known since the 1980s that such patients have an improved prognosis following coronary artery surgery if their disease is severe enough to warrant it.[24]

Exercise testing

Reversible myocardial ischaemia is looked for routinely by exercise testing (Fig. 6.8). The commonest practice in the UK is to use a graded incremental exercise protocol such as the Bruce protocol on a treadmill. Before referring a person for exercise testing, the doctor must consider whether he or she will be able to work hard enough to provide useful information about the heart. Individuals with lower limb or back arthritis, intermittent claudication or respiratory disease should be asked about their usual limiting factor during exercise.

> Individuals with lower limb or back arthritis, intermittent claudication or respiratory disease should be asked about their usual limiting factor during exercise

Reversible myocardial ischaemia is diagnosed from characteristic ECG changes which occur during exercise and revert to normal on recovery (Fig. 6.9). These changes cannot be analysed in the presence of a bundle branch block and are less reliable in patients with LVH or who are receiving digoxin therapy. In those

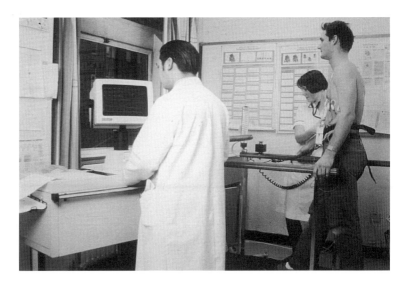

FIG. 6.8 Patient under-going treadmill exercise testing.

circumstances, a radioisotope myocardial perfusion scan should be requested.

Chronic heart failure is characterized by exercise intolerance. Traditional methods of classifying severity, such as the New York Heart Association system, rely on patients' subjective experience of their symptoms and exercise capacity. It is therefore useful to have an objective measure of exercise capacity by formal testing. A graded incremental treadmill test is of course an artificial situation

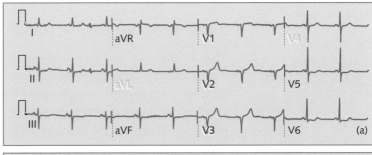

FIG. 6.9 Twelve lead ECGs from an exercise test showing significant ST depression during exercise. (a) At rest; (b) at peak exercise.

and does not recreate typical daily exercise. Other means of exercising have therefore been devised, including the 6-min walking test which involves the patient walking as far as possible on a measured track, for example a corridor, for 6 min. This can be performed without the need for expensive treadmill and monitoring equipment.

> The 6-min walking test can be performed without the need for expensive treadmill and monitoring equipment

Exercise capacity correlates poorly with measurements of central haemodynamics.[25] A better correlation with the severity of heart failure and prognosis is obtained with the maximum amount of oxygen the body can take up during exercise (peak Vo_2).[26] This requires a gas analyser to allow constant measurement of the concentrations of oxygen and carbon dioxide in the patient's breath during exercise. It is a reproducible parameter[27] and may be used to monitor the effects of drug therapy and to time the referral for cardiac transplantation in younger patients. However, the need for expensive equipment limits the use of this test to major cardiac centres. A useful surrogate is a treadmill test using the Standardized Exponential Exercise Protocol (STEEP), from which a measure of oxygen uptake may be derived.

> A measure of oxygen uptake may be derived from a treadmill test using the STEEP protocol

Radionuclide myocardial perfusion scanning

This is superior to other non-invasive tests for the detection, localization and grading of coronary artery disease. The functional information provided complements the anatomical information provided by coronary angiography. A radioactive tracer (usually thallium-201) is injected and taken up by metabolically active (and hence viable) myocardium in proportion to its perfusion. Injection of the tracer during stress brought about either by exercise or following the administration of a pharmacological agent such as dipyridamole shows an underperfused area of myocardium as an area of non-uptake. When scanned again after 4 h or more of rest, during which the isotope redistributes, these areas may image normally, indicating reversible ischaemia (Plate 6.2, facing p. 84). Myocardium which fails to take up the tracer at all at rest is considered to be infarcted and non-viable.

Unfortunately, this technique requires the administration of a considerable dose of radiation to the patient. It is also expensive to perform and takes about 4 h in total between the stress and resting images. Not every hospital has access to scanning facilities or the technical and medical experience to perform and interpret them.

Recently, the concept of hibernating myocardium[28] has come to the fore. We now know that abnormal left ventricular function at rest need not be due to irreversible myocardial necrosis. A segment showing systolic dysfunction on echocardiography or other imaging technique is usually due to irreversible scarring but may in some patients be due to viable, but dysfunctioning, myocardium. Myocardium which has chronically reduced perfusion may show down-regulation of metabolic and contractile function and be 'hibernating' as a protecting measure against necrosis. If the blood supply to that area of hibernating myocardium is restored early enough by revascularization, function may return either partially or completely, improving long-term survival.[29] Hibernating areas may be identified by their slow uptake of thallium at rest.

Hibernating areas may be identified by their slow uptake of thallium at rest

Coronary angiography and left ventriculography, and cardiac catheterization

This is the most invasive of routine cardiac investigations, but currently the only routine way to delineate the coronary artery anatomy (Fig. 6.10). It is usually reserved for patients with evidence of reversible ischaemia on either exercise testing or radionuclide scanning in whom coronary artery surgery is contemplated. In cases where other investigations have failed to show an aetiology for left ventricular dysfunction, it may be necessary to look for evidence of significant coronary artery disease by way of coronary angiography. A myocardial biopsy can also be taken in cases of suspected cardiomyopathy or myocarditis.

This is the most invasive of routine cardiac investigations, but currently the only routine way to delineate the coronary artery anatomy

Left ventricular function is routinely assessed before coronary

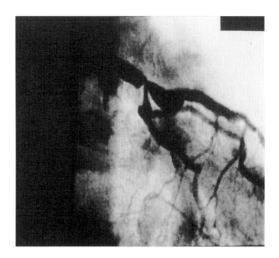

Fig. 6.10 Left main stem coronary artery stenosis on angiography.

angiography by means of single-plane contrast ventriculography and by direct measurement of the left ventricular end-diastolic pressure. Right and left heart catheterization may occasionally be used to provide important haemodynamic information, such as an accurate assessment of cardiac output and both systemic and pulmonary vascular resistance. Left-to-right shunts, for example atrial or ventricular septal defects, may be assessed by catheterization.

The major drawback is the invasive nature of the test. Each angiogram takes on average 40 min to perform and the patient, who is usually given some form of sedation, requires at least a day-case admission. Morbidity and a small mortality are associated with the procedure. For the most part, this takes the form of a small haematoma at the femoral arterial puncture site, but in a few cases more major complications can require urgent cardiac surgery.

24-h ambulatory ECG monitoring

This should be requested on any patient with heart failure who has a history of syncope or near syncope if routine electrocardiography does not provide diagnostic information. Treatable paroxysmal tachy- or bradyarrhythmias may be detected, but a single 24-h monitoring period may be insufficient to capture an infrequent arrhythmia. A cardio-memo recorder may be used to allow the patient to record a 30-s ECG during symptoms (provided the symptoms are not disabling).

24-h ambulatory ECG monitoring should be requested on any patient with heart failure who has a history of syncope or near syncope if routine ECG does not provide diagnostic information

Who should be referred?

Ideally, all patients with this potentially lethal cardiac condition should be seen by a cardiologist. Realistically, however, the size of the problem of heart failure means that if the health service is to investigate everybody adequately, the responsibility for doing so will lie primarily with the GP. There can be few hard and fast rules as to who should be referred on to a cardiology clinic for specialist assessment and management, and a GP should feel at liberty to refer anyone. However, as a suggested guideline, Table 6.4 lists the groups of individuals who warrant referral.

TABLE 6.4 Groups of patients who should be referred for specialist assessment.

Those with significant angina and left ventricular dysfunction under the age of 70 years where coronary revascularization may be an issue

Those with significant valvular disease

Those with hypertrophic cardiomyopathy

Those with severely impaired left ventricular function, e.g. ejection fraction below 20%. This is the group with the worst prognosis and the most to gain from specialist advice and management

Those with recent-onset atrial fibrillation where cardioversion to sinus rhythm may be considered

Those under the age of 60 years with left ventricular dysfunction

Those with significant peripheral vascular disease in whom the possibility of renal vascular disease requires to be excluded prior to commencement of an angiotensin-converting enzyme (ACE) inhibitor

Those who are hypotensive — systolic blood pressure <100 mmHg prior to commencing ACE inhibitors or those who have a low serum Na$^+$ (e.g. <130 mmol/l)

Others who, in the opinion of the referring doctor, stand to benefit from specialist investigation and management

Future developments

Natriuretic peptides

It has been established that everyone with left ventricular systolic dysfunction could benefit by receiving treatment with an ACE inhibitor.[21, 22] Although heart failure is a common condition[30] — and set to become more so in the coming decade — much of it is subclinical. There is therefore a growing awareness of the need to develop a simple screening test. Intense research is being focused on the atrial natriuretic peptides as potential blood markers of left ventricular dysfunction. Atrial natriuretic peptide, its subunits and brain natriuretic peptide, the best characterized peptides, are produced by the myocardium of the atria and the ventricles, respectively. In left ventricular dysfunction, they are found in the plasma in increasing amounts.[31]

It may well be that by itself, or in combination with another simple test such as ECG, the measurement of one or more natriuretic peptide will allow the primary care physician to identify individuals with a high probability of having left ventricular

TABLE 6.5 A simplified plan for the diagnosis of heart failure.			
Necessary	Opposes	Supports	Excludes alternatives
Symptoms of heart failure	Normal electrocardiogram	Improvement of symptoms in response to treatment	Biochemistry, urinalysis + haematology (renal disease, anaemia)
Abnormal cardiac function (usually by echocardiography)		Cardiomegaly on chest X-ray	Chest X-ray (lung disease)
		Reduced exercise test duration	Pulmonary function tests (lung disease)
		Elevated plasma atrial natriuretic peptide (under evaluation)	

From The Task Force on Heart Failure of the European Society of Cardiology[11] with permission.

dysfunction.[32] They can then be sent for echocardiography and further investigations as outlined above.

Conclusions

Given its poor prognosis, chronic heart failure is an important diagnosis to make correctly. It is inherently difficult to diagnose with any certainty on clinical grounds alone, but by following a simple and logical plan of investigation, as outlined above (and summarized in Table 6.5), the GP will in most cases be able correctly to identify those individuals with significant left ventricular systolic dysfunction. This, together with an assessment of concomitant disease affecting subsequent treatment, will allow for proper management.

References

1 McKee PA, Castell WP, McNamara PM, Kannel WB. The natural history of congestive heart failure: the Framingham study. *N Engl J Med* 1971; **285**: 1441.

2 Harlan WR, Oberman A, Grimm R, Rosati RA. Chronic congestive heart failure in coronary artery disease: clinical criteria. *Ann Intern Med* 1977; **86**: 133.

3 Carlson KJ, Lee DC-S, Goroll AH, Leahy M, Johnson RA. An analysis of physicians' reasons for prescribing long-term digitalis therapy in outpatients. *J Chronic Dis* 1985; **38**: 733.

4 Marantz PR, Tobin JN, Wasstertheil-Smoker S *et al*. Relationship between left ventricular systolic function and congestive heart failure diagnosed by clinical criteria. *Circulation* 1988; **77**: 607–612.

5 Gadsboll N, Hoilund-Carlsen PF, Nielsen GG *et al*. Symptoms and signs of heart failure in patients with myocardial infarction: reproducibility and relationship to chest X-ray, radionuclide ventriculography and right heart catheterisation. *Eur Heart J* 1989; **10**: 1017–1028.

6 Forrester JS, Diamond G, Chatterjee K *et al*. Medical therapy of acute myocardial infarction by application of haemodynamic subsets. *N Engl J Med* 1976; **295**: 1356–1362.

7 Stevenson LW, Perloff JK. The limited reliability of physical signs for estimating haemodynamics in chronic heart failure. *JAMA* 1989; **261**: 884–888.

8 Eagle KA, Quertermous T, Singer DE *et al*. Left ventricular ejection fraction: physician estimates compared with gated blood pool scan measurements. *Arch Intern Med* 1988; **148**: 882–885.

9 Dougherty AT, Nascarelli GV, Gray EL, Hicks CH, Goldstein RA. Congestive heart failure with normal systolic function. *Am J Cardiol* 1984; **54**: 778–782.

10 Clarkson P, Wheeldon NM, MacDonald TM. Left ventricular dysfunction. *Q J Med* 1994; **87**: 143–148.

11 The Task Force on Heart Failure of the European Society of Cardiology. Guidelines for the diagnosis of heart failure. *Eur Heart J* 1995; **16**: 741–751.

12 Iwasaki K, Kusachi S, Kazuyoshi H *et al*. Q-wave regression unrelated to patency of infarct-related artery or left ventricular ejection fraction or volume

after anterior wall acute myocardial infarction treated with or without reperfusion therapy. *Am J Cardiol* 1995; **78**: 14–20.

13 Myerburg RJ. Electrocardiography. In: Wilson JD, Braunwald E, Isselbacher KJ *et al*. (eds) *Harrison's Principles of Internal Medicine*, 12th edn. McGraw-Hill, New York, 1991.

14 Levy D, Garrison RJ, Savage DD, Kannel WB, Castelli WP. Left ventricular mass and incidence of coronary heart disease in an elderly cohort. The Framingham study. *Ann Intern Med* 1989; **110**: 101–107.

15 Hammond IW, Devereux RB, Alderman MH *et al*. The prevalence and correlates of echocardiographic left ventricular hypertrophy among employed patients with uncomplicated hypertension. *J Am Coll Cardiol* 1988; **7**: 639–650.

16 The Cardiac Arrhythmia Suppression Trial (CAST) Investigators. Preliminary report: effect of ecainide and flecainide on mortality in a randomised trial of arrhythmia suppression after myocardial infarction. *N Engl J Med* 1989; **321**: 406–412.

17 Armstrong P, Wastie ML. The heart. In: *Diagnostic Imaging*, 2nd edn. Blackwell Scientific Publications, Oxford, 1987.

18 Madsen EB, Gilpin E, Slutsky YA, Ahnve S, Henning H, Ross J. Usefulness of the chest X-ray for predicting abnormal left ventricular function after acute myocardial infarction. *Am Heart J* 1984, **108**: 1431–1436.

19 Gardin JM, Siscovick D, Anton-Culver H *et al*. Sex, age and disease affect echocardiographic left ventricular mass and systolic function in the free-living elderly. *Circulation* 1995; **91**: 1739–1748.

20 Cohn JN, Johnson GR, Shabetai R *et al*. for the V-HeFT VA Co-operative Studies Group. Ejection fraction, peak exercise oxygen consumption, cardiothoracic ratio, ventricular arrhythmias and plasma norepinephrine as determinants of prognosis in heart failure. *Circulation* 1993; **87**(suppl VI): V15–V16.

21 The SOLVD Investigators. Effect of enalapril on survival in patients with reduced left ventricular ejection fractions and congestive heart failure. *N Engl J Med* 1991; **325**: 293–302.

22 The SOLVD Investigators. Effect of enalapril on mortality and the development of heart failure in asymptomatic patients with reduced left ventricular ejection fractions. *N Engl J Med* 1992; **327**: 685–691.

23 Beming J, Rokkedal Nielsen J, Launbjerg J, Fogh J, Mickley H, Andersen PE. Rapid estimation of left ventricular ejection fraction in acute myocardial infarction by echocardiographic wall motion analysis. *Cardiology* 1992; **80**: 257–266.

24 Alderman EL, Fisher LD, Litwin P *et al*. Results of coronary artery surgery in patients with poor left ventricular function (CASS). *Circulation* 1983; **68**: 785–795.

25 Wilson JR, Rayos G, Yroh TK, Gothard P, Bak K. Dissociation between exertional symptoms and circulatory failure in patients with heart failure. *Circulation* 1995; **92**: 47–53.

26 Parameshwar J, Keegan J, Sparrow H, Sutton GC, Poole-Wilson PA. Predictors of prognosis in severe chronic heart failure. *Am Heart J* 1992; **123**: 421–426.

27 Lipkin DP, Perrins J, Poole-Wilson PA. Respiratory gas exchange in the assessment of patients with impaired ventricular function. *Br Heart J* 1985; **54**: 321–328.

28 Rahimtoola SH. A perspective on the three large multicentre randomised clinical trials of coronary bypass surgery for chronic stable angina. *Circulation* 1985; **72–V**: 123.

29 Pigott JD, Kouchonos NT, Oberman A, Cutter GR. Late results of surgical and medical therapy for patients with coronary artery disease and depressed left ventricular function. *J Am Coll Cardiol* 1985; **5**: 10–45.

30 Kannel WB, Ho K, Thom T. Changing epidemiological features of cardiac failure. *Br Heart J* 1994; **72**(suppl): S3–S9.

31 Burnett JC, Kao PC, Hu DC *et al.* Atrial natriuretic peptide elevation in congestive heart failure in the human. *Science* 1986; **231**: 1145–1147.

32 Lerman A, Gibbons RJ, Rodeheffer RJ *et al.* Circulating N-terminal ANP as a marker for symptomless left ventricular dysfunction. *Lancet* 1993; **341**: 1105–1108.

Diuretics in Chronic Heart Failure

SUMMARY POINTS

- Diuretic efficacy is often reduced in chronic heart failure and more regular dosing or a combination of diuretics is sometimes required
- Thiazides have been replaced by loop diuretics as first-line diuretics for heart failure
- Metolazone is effective in patients with renal dysfunction
- Hyponatraemia and hypokalaemia are common problems with the use of diuretics in chronic heart failure
- Diuretics interact with a number of different drugs, including non-steroidal anti-inflammatory drugs, vasodilators and digoxin
- Patients may have to organize their day around the period of most intense diuresis

The introduction of powerful oral diuretics represented a major advance in the management of chronic heart failure (CHF). Indeed, five decades were to pass before the next major breakthrough — the use of angiotensin-converting enzyme (ACE) inhibitors. Despite the rapid uptake of these newer drugs and the spread of their use to all classes of symptomatic heart failure, diuretics remain a mainstay of the treatment. It has been clearly shown that once the requirement for diuretics has been demonstrated, no other class of drugs is as effective at combating fluid retention.[1]

> Once the requirement for diuretics has been demonstrated, no other class of drugs is as effective at combating fluid retention

Powerful orally active diuretics were welcomed by both patients and their doctors because of their marked symptomatic benefits. The cosmetic effect of removing oedema was also important as a sign that the patient was improving. It could be argued that this merely removed the offending signs of heart failure and did nothing for the heart disease itself, thereby engendering a false sense of security in the patient and optimism in the doctor. However, although there are no studies of the impact of diuretics on survival in heart failure, situations of severe fluid retention would be unlikely to resolve as well without diuretics, even though acute heart failure may respond as well to careful vasodilator therapy.[2]

Today, with the judicious use of intravenous or oral diuretics, often in combination and accompanied by restriction of fluid intake, refractory oedema has become uncommon. Nevertheless, at this stage, diuretics could be said to be merely palliative as a very advanced stage of the underlying heart disease will have been reached.

The main types of diuretics, their sites of action in the nephron and their potency are summarized in Table 7.1. Broadly, there are three main groups:
- powerful loop diuretics (such as frusemide and bumetanide);
- moderately potent and older drugs (thiazides);
- weak diuretics acting at the distal tubule.

All directly or indirectly reduce sodium reabsorption and thereby lead to increased urinary output.

TABLE 7.1 Summary of main types of diuretics, their site of action and potency.

Diuretic	Site of action	Filtered sodium excretion (%)
Potent Frusemide Bumetanide	Loop of Henle	15–25%
Moderate Thiazides Metolazone	Cortical diluting segment	5–10%
Weak Spironolactone Amiloride	Distal tubule	1–5%

Loop diuretics

The only commonly used agents in this class are frusemide and bumetanide. They act by blocking active chloride transport from the lumen of the ascending limb of the loop of Henle into the blood stream;[3] sodium and water are also retained in the lumen, to maintain ionic and osmotic balance. About 25% of all the sodium and water filtered at the glomerulus is reabsorbed in this part of the tubule. As about 180 l/day is filtered into the renal tubules, the potential in terms of urinary output of even only partially blocking 25% of that amount is clearly colossal in volume terms.

The effective dose of frusemide is usually 40 mg (equivalent to 1 mg bumetanide). However, a dose as high as 80–120 mg may be necessary as there is often reduced diuretic efficiency in CHF. If a greater diuretic response is needed, repeated rather than larger doses should be used. Rarely, a very high dose (up to 4000 mg/day) frusemide may be required in refractory CHF, particularly if there is significant renal dysfunction.[4] It is our preferred approach to add another diuretic with a different nephron site of action before increasing the dose of frusemide above 120 mg twice daily.

> It is our preferred approach to add another diuretic with a different nephron site of action before increasing the dose of frusemide above 120 mg twice daily

Thiazide diuretics

Thiazide diuretics are firmly established in the treatment of hypertension, but have largely been supplanted by loop diuretics as first-line drugs in the management of heart failure.

The cortical diluting segment of the nephron is responsible for reabsorbing 10–15% of the filtered load of sodium, explaining why thiazides which act there are significantly less potent than drugs acting on the loop of Henle.[5] The fact that their action is more evenly spread over 24 h is advantageous in terms of a less abrupt action, but disadvantageous in terms of causing more nocturia.

In practice, thiazides (for example, bendrofluazide 5–10 mg) are usually used in addition to loop diuretics in the treatment of resistant CHF; however, it may be possible in cases of mild fluid retention, particularly in patients willing to live on a restricted fluid intake, to use thiazides as first-line agents.

Combining loop diuretics and thiazides is effective,[6] but should be used with great care as unpredictably large diuretic effects may occur, leading to intravascular dehydration, hypotension, severe electrolyte upset (particularly hyponatraemia) and renal failure. Thiazides are ineffective in renal failure.[7]

> Combining loop diuretics and thiazides is effective, but should be used with great care as unpredictably large diuretic effects may occur

Metolazone

Metolazone resembles the thiazides and probably acts chiefly at the same region of the nephron. However, it does have some action on the proximal tubule. Although this is mild, the fact that the proximal tubule is responsible for reabsorbing 60–70% of the 180 l filtered at the glomerulus each day means that even a weak action may have a considerable effect.[7] For this reason, metolazone is considered to be of intermediate potency between the thiazides and the loop diuretics. Perhaps even greater care has to be exercised when using it in combination with a loop diuretic, as that entails impairing sodium and water reabsorption at three sites in the nephron. The combination is considered the most potent of any two diuretics currently available.

Unlike the thiazides, metolazone remains effective in patients with renal impairment of at least moderate severity, offering greater flexibility of management in that group of patients.[8]

> Unlike the thiazides, metolazone remains effective in patients with renal impairment of at least moderate severity, offering greater flexibility of management

Potassium-sparing diuretics

These drugs, principally spironolactone and amiloride, act on the mechanisms in the distal tubule whereby sodium is reabsorbed in exchange for potassium or hydrogen, thus conserving potassium while eliminating sodium. As potassium loss is an inevitable result of delivering more sodium to this region of the tubule, where it is normally reabsorbed in exchange for potassium, this type of diuretic would seem almost optimal. However, the sodium-losing effect is quite weak and, in practice, these drugs are usually used in association with the more potent loop or thiazide diuretics; spironolactone is more often used on its own than amiloride.

Spironolactone is a competitive aldosterone inhibitor. Amiloride acts independently of aldosterone to prevent sodium–potassium exchange in the distal nephron (all three agents also prevent H⁺ loss, which also reduces K⁺ loss). These drugs are, by themselves, weak natriuretics and enhance the sodium-losing effects of other diuretics when given in combination; there is also a report that spironolactone and captopril in combination may induce natriuresis in resistant CHF.

> There is a report that spironolactone and captopril in combination may induce natriuresis in resistant CHF

Adverse effects of diuretics

Hyponatraemia

Hyponatraemia is a limiting factor in diuretic therapy and a common clinical sign indicating a poor prognosis.[9]

Complex intrarental mechanisms explain in part the fall in plasma sodium that occurs in many patients with severe heart failure receiving regular diuretic therapy.[10] They include the direct effects of angiotensin II and antidiuretic hormone, which are both elevated in severe heart failure, particularly in patients receiving diuretics.[11] Other simpler causes include the thirst that patients experience with diuretics, causing them to drink more water. As the fluid lost as a result of diuretic administration contains sodium, it is not surprising that dilutional hyponatraemia is common even when total body sodium remains increased, as in patients with resistant oedema.

> As the fluid lost as a result of diuretic administration contains sodium, it is not surprising that dilutional hyponatraemia is common even when total body sodium remains increased

In less severe heart failure, particularly among elderly patients, even thiazides can cause hyponatraemia, especially when combined with amiloride; however, it is usually reversible with reduction in dose of diuretic and/or fluid intake.

In patients with heart failure, hyponatraemia usually indicates marked stimulation of the renin–angiotensin system, often accompanied by hypokalaemia.[12] Great care must be taken when starting ACE inhibitors in this situation, and hospital supervision is indicated.

Mild hyponatraemia is almost universal in patients with moderate or severe heart failure treated with diuretics. Clinically, the only way of managing hyponatraemia, or preventing its development, is to institute some degree of fluid restriction, especially in patients with marked oedema receiving high doses of diuretics. Greater fluid restriction (1–1.5 l/day) is essential when the plasma sodium concentration falls below 130 mmol/l. In the most severe cases of hyponatraemia, haemoperfusion or peritoneal dialysis may be required to correct this and other electrolyte abnormalities. As total body sodium is elevated in these patients, it seems illogical to correct a maldistribution of sodium and water with an infusion of sodium solutions.

> Mild hyponatraemia is almost universal in patients with moderate or severe heart failure treated with diuretics

Potassium

Like sodium, most of the potassium filtered at the glomerulus is reabsorbed in the proximal tubule; much of the potassium excreted results from secretion in the distal convoluted tubule in exchange for reabsorbed sodium. The extent of this exchange depends on several factors, including:
- acid–base status (hydrogen may also exchange with sodium);
- distal delivery of sodium and potassium;
- plasma levels of aldosterone.

Both loop diuretics and thiazides cause potassium depletion, to which patients with CHF are already predisposed as a result of neuroendocrine activation. Potassium deficiency increases the risk of digitalis toxicity (and toxicity from other potentially arrhythmogenic drugs such as tricyclic antidepressants, pheno-thiazines and antiarrhythmic agents). Hypokalaemia may also directly predispose to serious ventricular arrhythmias. There is thus a strong case for avoiding potassium depletion in patients with CHF. Diuretic therapy may influence body potassium directly or through stimulation of the renin–angiotensin system, although there has been considerable controversy on the latter point. Low-dose diuretic therapy does not cause total body potassium depletion in patients who are eating a diet rich in potassium.[13] Although this may be the case in patients with mild heart failure, these findings have not been confirmed in several studies of patients with severe heart failure.[14]

> Diuretic therapy may influence body potassium directly or through stimulation of the renin–angiotensin system

Hyperkalaemia can also occur with the use of potassium-conserving diuretics, especially in the elderly. This is primarily a risk in patients with impaired renal function or diabetes mellitus, and in those taking other drugs such as potassium supplements, ACE inhibitors or non-steroidal anti-inflammatory drugs (NSAIDs).

Magnesium depletion is common in diuretic-treated CHF patients and has similar adverse effects to potassium depletion. It may be impossible to correct potassium deficiency unless magnesium deficiency is corrected first. Potassium-conserving diuretics also conserve magnesium.

Interactions

NSAIDs blunt the natriuretic effect of diuretics by poorly understood and possible different mechanisms. NSAIDs may also cause renal dysfunction and hyperkalaemia in patients treated with potassium supplements, potassium-conserving diuretics and ACE inhibitors. This is a particular concern in the elderly.

Hyperkalaemia due to the combination of an ACE inhibitor and a potassium-conserving diuretic may occur, although in our practice it appears to be much less common than expected; an ACE inhibitor alone may be insufficient to prevent electrolyte depletion.

Vasodilators

Chronic diuretic treatment may activate vasoconstrictor neurohumoral systems, but appears to enhance arterial vasodilator responsiveness in oedematous patients. The theory that diuretics contribute to progression of CHF by causing adverse neurohumoral changes may therefore be too simplistic.

> The theory that diuretics contribute to progression of CHF by causing adverse neurohumoral changes may be too simplistic

Digoxin

Clearly, diuretic-induced hypokalaemia may predispose to digoxin toxicity, leading primarily to arrhythmia. This can be avoided by regular — not necessarily frequent — checks on the patient's urea and electrolyte status to ensure that hypokalaemia is detected and treated and that renal impairment is not developing. This is especially important as all patients requiring diuretic therapy should also receive an ACE inhibitor.

Neuroendocrine stimulation

In addition to electrolyte abnormalities, all types of diuretics cause neuroendocrine stimulation. Frusemide has been shown to cause both acute and chronic stimulation of the sympathetic nervous system and the renin–angiotensin–aldosterone system. Acute stimulation is associated with a sharp increase in systemic vascular resistance. These potentially adverse neuroendocrine and haemodynamic changes can be countered by treatment with an ACE inhibitor.

Other important adverse effects include hyperuricaemia, which may be only too obvious with the development of gout, of which by far the commonest cause is diuretic therapy. Acute gout should be treated in the usual way with an effective anti-inflammatory, followed by allopurinol to lower the uric acid level in the blood if a reduction in diuretics is not possible, as is usually the case. Obviously, closer monitoring of the renal function and electrolytes will be necessary if a potent NSAID is used.

A potentially more hazardous and often less clinically obvious side-effect of diuretics is glucose intolerance leading to frank clinical diabetes. This should be considered when no obvious reason for a decrease in well-being occurs, even in the absence of more obvious clinical clues to the onset of diabetes. Again, little can be done since diuretic therapy cannot usually be withdrawn. There is some evidence that bumetanide might cause slightly less glucose intolerance than frusemide but, once it has developed, it does not usually resolve on switching therapy.

> Diabetes should be considered when no obvious reason for a decrease in well-being occurs even in the absence of more obvious clinical clues

Practical points

The spectrum of use and range of diuretic dosage in heart failure is wide: for example, from 6 mg of bendrofluazide on alternate days to 1 g/day frusemide, according to individual practice or as part of a planned therapeutic strategy of increasing complexity. It is worth emphasizing that, in the absence of a contraindication, all patients requiring a diuretic for heart failure must also be treated with an ACE inhibitor. Many patients with mild symptoms can be managed with a thiazide diuretic, but most patients will eventually graduate to the more potent loop diuretics, frusemide or bumetanide.

> In the absence of a contraindication, all patients requiring a diuretic for heart failure must also be treated with an ACE inhibitor

As a general rule, if monotherapy with frusemide (80 mg/day) is not effective, the use of vasodilator therapy should be considered. In refractory patients, increasing doses of potent diuretics may be complemented by the addition of a thiazide or metolazone. In the absence of an ACE inhibitor, the further addition of a potassium-conserving agent, such as amiloride, spironolactone or triamterene, completes the triple theory approach to diuretic treatment. For clinical purposes, there is little to choose among the members of each diuretic class, and individual usage varies widely.

> For clinical purposes, there is little to choose among the members of each diuretic class, and individual usage varies widely

All diuretics cause inconvenience for patients, who usually have to organize their daily activities around the period of most intense diuresis. Loop diuretics may often be preferred as their effect generally diminishes 4 h after the dose. Patients should, of course, be informed that there is generally no fixed time of day that diuretics must be taken and, according to individual circumstances, the dose may be taken in the morning, afternoon or evening (but not too late, as the diuresis may interrupt sleep).

Patients may also be flexible with regard to the diuretic dose. Ours are instructed to record their daily weight (on rising, after voiding, before breakfast) and, if there is a consistent (more than 3 consecutive days) increase of more than 0.5 kg, they are advised to increase the diuretic dose until 'dry weight' is regained. For example, a patient receiving 40 mg frusemide who puts on weight unexpectedly (or who feels more breathless, develops ankle swelling, etc.) would be advised to take an extra frusemide tablet (increasing the dose from 40 to 80 mg) for up to a week. If there was no response within a week, or if the weight gain or symptoms worsened, the patient should be instructed to seek medical help.

References

1 Richardson A, Bayliss J, Scriven AJ, Parameshwar J, Poole-Wilson PA, Sutton GC. Double-blind comparison of captopril alone against frusemide plus amiloride in mild heart failure. *Br Heart J* 1987; **57**: 80–84.

2 Nelson GIC, Silke B, Ahuja RC, Hussain M, Taylor SH. Haemodynamic advantages of isosorbide dinitrate over frusemide in acute heart failure following myocardial infarction. *Lancet* 1983; **i**: 730–733.

3 Burg MB, Green N. Function of the thick ascending limb of the loop of Henle. *Am J Physiol* 1973; **224**: 659–668.

4 Kuchar DL, O'Rourke MF. High-dose frusemide in refractory cardiac failure. *Eur Heart J* 1985; **6**: 954–958.

5 Masterson BJ, Epstein M. Thiazide diuretics, chlortalidone, and metolazone. In: Messerli HF (ed) *Cardiovascular Drug Therapy*. WB Saunders, Philadelphia, 1990, pp 337–347.

6 Channer KS, Richardson M, Crook R, Jones JV. Thiazides with loop diuretics for severe congestive heart failure. *Lancet* 1990; **1**: 922–923.

7 Reubi F, Cotter P. Effects of reduced glomerular filtration rate on responsiveness to chlorothiazide and diuretics. *Circulation* 1965; **23**: 200.

8 Dargie HJ, Allison MEM, Kennedy AC, Gray MHJ. High-dose metolazone in chronic renal failure. *Br Med J* 1972; **4**: 196.

9 Lee WH, Packer M. Prognostic importance of serum sodium concentration and its modification by converting enzyme inhibition in patients with severe chronic heart failure. *Circulation* 1986; **73**: 257–267.

10 Gross P, Ketteler M, Hausmann C *et al.* Role of diuretics, hormonal derangements, and clinical setting of hyponatremia in medical patients. *Klin Wochenschr* 1988; **66**: 662–669.

11 Nader PC, Thompson JR, Alpern RJ. Complications of diuretic use. *Semin Nephrol* 1988; **8**: 365–370.

12 Dargie HJ. Interrelation of electrolytes and renin–angiotensin system in congestive heart failure. *Am J Cardiol* 1990; **65**(suppl): 28E–32E.

13 Dargie HJ, Boddy K, Kennedy AC, King PC, Read PR, Ward DM. Total body potassium on long-term frusemide therapy: is potassium supplementation necessary? *Br Med J* 1974; **4**: 316–319.

14 Lawson DH, O'Conner PC. Drug-attributed alterations in potassium handling in congestive heart failure. *Eur J Clin Pharmacol* 1982; **23**: 21–25.

Treatment of Heart Failure: ACE Inhibitors

SUMMARY POINTS

• Angiotensin-converting enzyme inhibitors have been shown to improve prognosis in all degrees of left ventricular dysfunction

• These drugs have their effect by inhibiting the production of angiotensin II which consequently affects blood vessels, kidneys and the heart, and is also thought to interact with the sympathetic and parasympathetic nervous systems

• Continuing treatment is required to maintain the benefit of angiotensin-converting enzyme inhibitors on disease control

• In cases of severe, moderate and mild left ventricular dysfunction, the use of angiotensin-converting enzyme inhibitors reduces the need for hospital admission

• Studies have shown that angiotensin-converting enzyme inhibitors cause a highly significant reduction in mortality

• The side-effect profile for angiotensin-converting enzyme inhibitors includes first-dose hypotension, long-term dizziness and hypotension, renal dysfunction, hyperkalaemia and cough, although these are relatively infrequent and rarely troublesome

Since their development two decades ago, angiotensin-converting enzyme (ACE) inhibitors have become the mainstay of treatment of patients with left ventricular dysfunction. Unlike any other treatment, they improve prognosis in all cases, whether acute or chronic, symptomatic or asymptomatic.

How do ACE inhibitors work in heart failure?

ACE inhibitors reverse many of the pathophysiological abnormalities that characterize heart failure (Fig. 8.1).[1,2] Their primary effect is to inhibit production of the hormone angiotensin II, which has multiple direct and indirect actions on the blood vessels, kidneys and heart (Fig. 8.2). Angiotensin II may also augment the activity of the sympathetic nervous system and inhibit

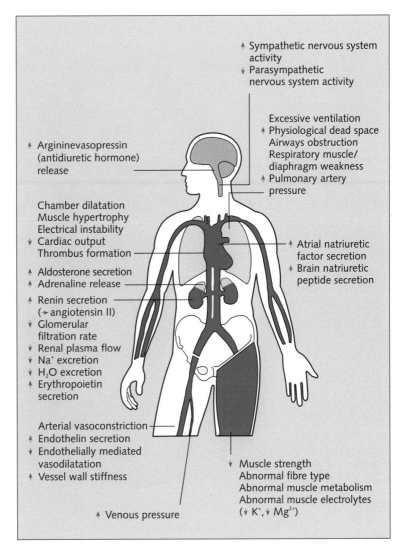

FIG. 8.1 Whilst the primary problem in chronic heart failure is cardiac, the clinical syndrome is characterized by secondary multi-system dysfunction.

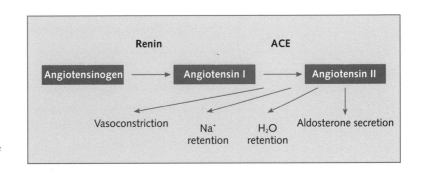

FIG. 8.2 The renin angiotensin aldosterone system.

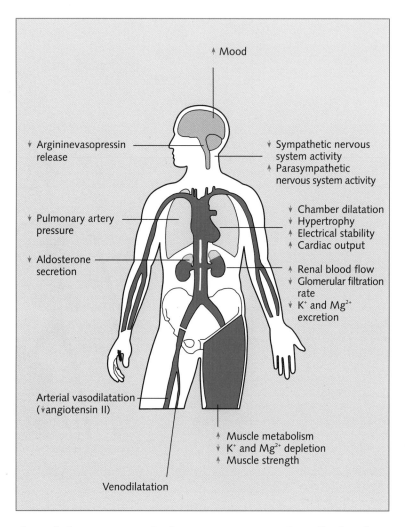

FIG. 8.3 Beneficial actions of ACE inhibitors in chronic heart failure; ACE inhibitors are not merely arterial and venous vasodilators.

that of the parasympathetic nervous system. Overall, therefore, ACE inhibitors act as mixed arterial and venous vasodilators, reversing the vasoconstriction that is such an important hallmark of heart failure, and unloading the heart. The major clinical consequence is an increase in skeletal muscle blood flow — an essential prerequisite for improved exercise capacity.

> ACE inhibitors act as mixed arterial and venous vasodilators, reversing vasoconstriction and unloading the heart

ACE inhibitors also have important effects on the kidneys, neurohormonal pathways, blood and cellular chemistry, and the electrical stability of the heart (Fig. 8.3). Through these and other mechanisms, they prevent further deterioration in cardiac function and progression of the heart failure state.

Evidence of benefit

Signs and symptoms

ACE inhibitors are used as an adjunct to diuretics in heart failure, not as a substitute or an alternative.[1-5] Numerous small and large studies have shown that ACE inhibitors used in this way reduce the symptoms of breathlessness and fatigue in patients with heart failure, producing a corresponding improvement in exercise tolerance and functional class (Fig. 8.4).[1,2] Signs of overt heart failure are also reduced (Fig. 8.4). These benefits are seen across all grades of heart failure, although improvement may take up to 3 months to become fully apparent.[1,2]

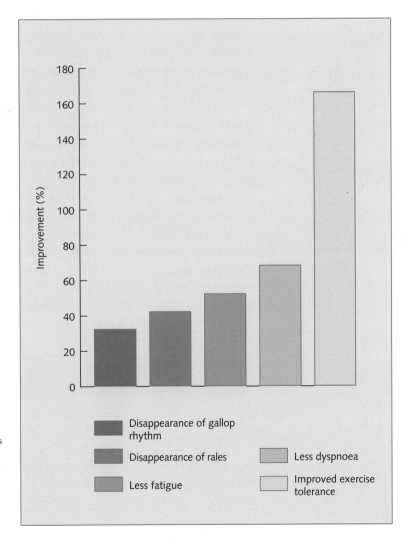

FIG. 8.4 Beneficial effects of enalapril on signs, symptoms and functional capacity in chronic heart failure compared with a placebo group. (After Giles 1990.)

109

Importantly, ACE inhibitors are more effective than other vasodilators at relieving symptoms.[3-5] They are also superior to digoxin.[6] However, other advantages also explain why ACE inhibitors have become the bedrock of the treatment of heart failure.

> ACE inhibitors are more effective than other vasodilators at relieving symptoms. They are also superior to digoxin

Progression of heart failure

When left unchecked, heart failure tends to be a relentlessly progressive syndrome. Patients initially classified as having mild heart failure deteriorate over time, eventually developing severe disease; in other words, they progress from New York Heart Association (NYHA) class II to class IV. As the syndrome worsens, quality of life deteriorates, hospitalization becomes more frequent and treatment costs rise.

Several studies have shown that early initiation of ACE inhibitor therapy slows disease progression. The best illustration of this comes from the Munich Mild Heart Failure Trial (Fig. 8.5).[7] In this study, over a median follow-up period of 2–7 years, only 11% of patients treated with the ACE inhibitor captopril progressed from NYHA class II to class IV, as compared to 26% of placebo treated patients. The benefit to any individual patient of remaining in NYHA class II and experiencing only slight limitation of ordinary activities, compared with progressing to class IV and experiencing dyspnoea and other symptoms at rest, should not be underestimated. It is also important to emphasize that continuing treatment is required to maintain continuing benefit. Withdrawal of treatment results in deterioration of the heart failure state (Fig. 8.6).[8]

> Several studies have shown that early initiation of ACE inhibitor therapy slows disease progression

Hospitalization

One poorly recognized benefit of ACE inhibitors in patients with left ventricular dysfunction is that they reduce the need for hospital admission for heart failure. This has been one of the most

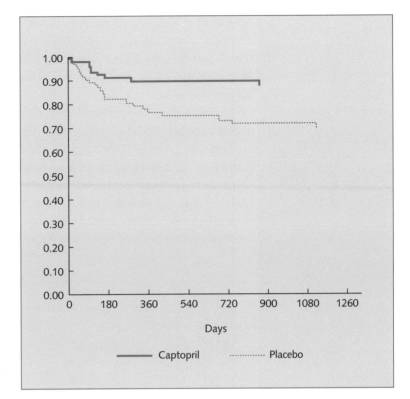

FIG. 8.5 Survival time analysis (Kaplan–Meier) for the end-point 'progression of heart failure to NYHA class IV on optimal adjusted therapy'. (From Kleber *et al.* 1992.[7])

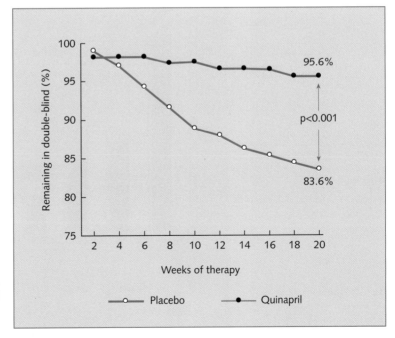

FIG. 8.6 Cumulative percentage of patients withdrawing from double-blind treatment because of lack of efficacy. (From Pflugfelder *et al.* 1993.[8])

111

consistently demonstrated effects of ACE inhibitors and is observed in studies of patients with severe, moderate, mild and even asymptomatic disease (Fig. 8.7). It reflects the ability of ACE inhibitors to reduce symptoms and signs and retard or prevent progression of heart failure.

Once again the magnitude of benefit should not be underestimated. For example, in the treatment arm of the Studies of Left Ventricular Dysfunction (SOLVD), the largest trial performed to date in patients with heart failure, ACE inhibition reduced hospitalization rates by 30%.[10] In absolute terms, enalapril therapy resulted in 67 fewer hospitalizations for heart failure (and 100 fewer total hospitalizations) per 1000 patient-years of treatment (that is, for example, treating 200 patients for

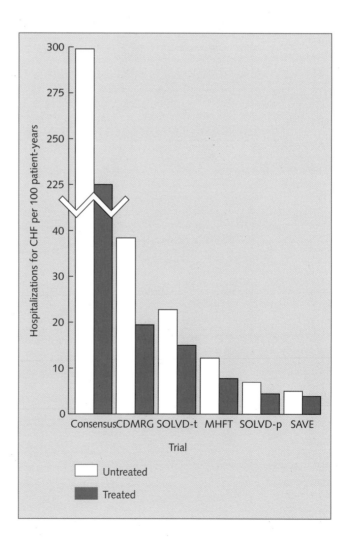

FIG. 8.7 Hospitalizations for CHF per 100 patient-years. (From McMurray & Davie, 1996.[9])

5 years). This difference was observed despite survival of more patients in the enalapril group than in the placebo group.

This is an extremely important benefit for the individual patient and society as a whole. A person with heart failure has a 20–30% chance of hospitalization in any given year. Furthermore, once a patient has deteriorated sufficiently to require hospitalization, mortality is high and the case fatality rate during hospitalization is to the order of 20%. In most ageing western societies, hospitalization for heart failure is a common and increasing problem; hospital admissions are not only numerous, but also prolonged and expensive.

A person with heart failure has a 20–30% chance of hospitalization within any given year

Mortality

The biggest breakthrough in the treatment of heart failure was the demonstration that mortality can be reduced if vasodilators and ACE inhibitors are given in addition to diuretics and digoxin. Prior to this, mortality from heart failure had remained appallingly and stubbornly high.

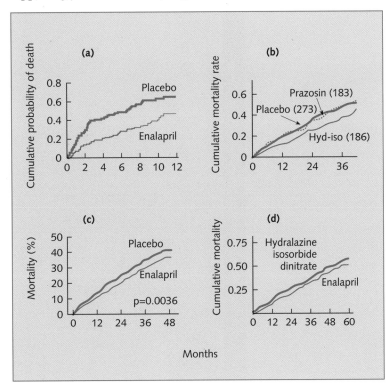

FIG. 8.8 Relative mortality rates of drugs in the major CHF studies. (a) CONSENSUS I; (b) V-HeFT I; (c) SOLVD (T); (d) V-HEFT II.

TABLE 8.1 Breakdown of treatment groups in recent CHF studies.

	V-HeFT I[11]			CONSENSUS I[12]		SOLVD(T)[10]		V-HeFT II[4]	
	Placebo	Prazosin	H-ISDN	Placebo	Enalapril	Placebo	Enalapril	HISDN	Enalapril
$n =$	273	183	186	126	127	1284	1285	401	403
Mean age (years)	59	58	58	70	71	61	61	61	61
Male (%)	100	100	100	71	70	80	81	100	100
NYHA II	—	—	—	0	0	57	57	52	50
III	—	—	—	0	0	31	30	42	44
IV	—	—	—	100	100	2	2	0.5	0.2
LVEF	30	29	30	—	—	25	25	29	29
IHD	44	44	44	74	72	72	70	52	54
Hypertension	43	40	40	19	24	42	43	45	50
Mean follow-up (months)		27.6			6.5		41.4		30.0

n, subjects enrolled in each treatment group; H-ISDN, combination treatment with hydralazine and isosorbide dinitrate; NYHA, New York Heart Association classification; LVEF, left ventricular ejection fraction; IHD, ischaemic heart disease; V-HeFT I, First Vasodilator Heart Failure Trial; V-HeFT II, Second Vasodilator Heart Failure Trial; CONSENSUS I, Co-operative North Scandanavian Enalapril Survival Study; SOLVD(T), Treatment of the Studies of Left Ventricular Dysfunction.

Four major mortality trials have been conducted with vasodilators in patients with overt clinical heart failure (Fig. 8.8 and Table 8.1). In 1986, the first Vasodilator Heart Failure Trial (VHeFT I) showed that the combination of hydralazine and isosorbide dinitrate (H-ISDN) appeared to improve prognosis when given in addition to conventional therapy; prazosin was no better than placebo.[11] The reduction in mortality seen in these patients with mild-to-moderate heart failure was, however, of borderline statistical significance and the treatment combination of H-ISDN was poorly tolerated. In 1987, CONSENSUS I showed a substantial and statistically highly significant reduction in mortality with adjunctive enalapril treatment in patients with very severe heart failure.[12]

Although clearly an impressive effect, it was not known whether benefit would also be seen in patients with lesser degrees of heart failure. When the treatment arm of SOLVD was published in 1991,[10] it showed that ACE inhibitors also reduced mortality in patients with mild and moderately severe heart failure, and produced a sizeable and highly statistically significant benefit. Finally, VHeFT II, a head-to-head comparison between H-ISDN and enalapril, reported that mortality was 28% lower in class II/III patients who received enalapril (mortality 32.8%) than in those treated with H-ISDN (mortality 38.2%) after 2 years of follow-up ($P = 0.016$).[4] Overall, enalapril resulted in 22 fewer premature deaths per 1000 patient-years of treatment than H-ISDN — a clinically substantial and meaningful advantage.

> Enalapril resulted in 22 fewer premature deaths per 1000 patient-years of treatment than H-ISDN — a clinically substantial and meaningful advantage

What does the mortality reduction with ACE inhibitors really mean?

It is often difficult to appreciate what a 16% relative reduction in mortality or a 4% absolute difference in event rates means in real terms. Table 8.2 tries to put CONSENSUS I and SOLVD into some sort of perspective, comparing the benefit in these trials to that obtained with other cardiovascular treatments. An alternative and valuable way of assessing the benefit of therapies is to use the 'number needed to treat' concept, shown in Table 8.3. Finally, it is also worth considering what the public health benefits of applying clinical trials to clinical practice might be.

115

TABLE 8.2 Benefits of ACE inhibitors in CHF in context.	
Treatment	Benefit: events prevented per 1000 patient-years of treatment
Diuretic/beta-blocker for mild hypertension	1–2 strokes
Aspirin after myocardial infarction	16 deaths/MI/strokes
Oral beta-blockers after myocardial infarction	13 deaths/5 MI
ACE inhibitor after myocardial infarction (low LVEF-SAVE)	12 deaths/9 MI/16 CHF/ 10 revascularizations
HMG CoA reductase inhibitor after myocardial infarction/angina (45)	6 deaths/12 MI/4CHF/ 11 revascularizations
ACE inhibitor for severe CHF	160 deaths
ACE inhibitor for mild/moderate CHF	16 deaths/3 MI — unstable angina 116 hospitalizations

CHF, chronic heart failure; LVEF, left ventricular ejection fraction; MI, myocardial infarction; SAVE, Survival and Ventricular Enlargement Study.

However one looks at these trials, it is clear that the benefit of ACE inhibitors in all grades of heart failure is substantial and worthwhile.

However one looks at these trials, it is clear that the benefit of ACE inhibitors in all grades of heart failure is substantial and worthwhile

The importance of using the right dose of ACE inhibitor

A common misconception about the use of ACE inhibitors relates to dosing. The doses prescribed in clinical practice are usually much smaller than those used in clinical trials, yet only the trial doses are known to be of benefit (Table 8.4). Indeed, there is other evidence to suggest that larger doses are more beneficial, and one study showed a clear dose–response relationship for quinapril with regard to improvement in exercise capacity. At present, it appears that doses similar to those used in clinical trials are necessary to ensure maximum clinical benefit. Administration of smaller doses may expose patients to the same potential adverse effects without the same potential benefit.

TABLE 8.3 Treatment benefits in cardiovascular disease.		
Treatment Severe CHF†	Events prevented Death	Patients treated for 1–2 years
Hypertension (DBP 115–129)	Death, CVA, MI	3
CABG for LMS stenosis	Death	3
Warfarin for AF (secondary prevention)	CVA	3
ACE inhibitor — heart failure post-MI**	Death, MI, CVA, CHF	4
ASA for TIA	Death, CVA	6
Warfarin for AF (primary prevention)	CVA	7
ACE inhibitor for mild CHF	CV death, hospital (CHF)	8
ACE inhibitor for LV* dysfunction post-MI	CV death, hospital (CHF)	10
HMG-CoA reductase inhibitor post-MI	CV death, MI, cardiac arrest	11
Aspirin post-MI	CV death, MI, CVA	12
Hypertension (DBP 90–109)	Death, CVA, MI	141

*Based on SAVE study.
** Based on AIRE study.
†Based on CONSENSUS I.
CV, cardiovascular; MI, myocardial infarction; ASA, aspirin; DBP, diastolic blood pressure; AF, atrial fibrillation; LV, left ventricular; TIA, transient ischaemic attack; CVA, cerebrovascular accident; CABG, coronary artery bypass grafting; LMS, left main stem coronary artery; hosp (CHF), hospitalization for chronic heart failure; AIRE, Acute Infarction Ramipril Efficacy Study.

It appears that doses similar to those used in clinical trials are necessary to ensure maximum clinical benefit

Adverse effects: the true picture

Perhaps the greatest misconception about ACE inhibitors relates to their side-effect profile. Few classes of drugs have acquired such an unwarranted reputation for adverse effects as ACE inhibitors, although few drugs have had so many thousands of patient-years of placebo-controlled observations to give a true picture of tolerability.

TABLE 8.4 Effective dose of ACE inhibitors.

Trial	ACE inhibitor	Target dose	Mean daily dose
Symptoms/exercise time			
Captopril Multicenter			
Research Group 1983	Captopril	100 mg tds	221 mg
Cleland *et al.* 1984	Captopril	50 mg tds	93.75 mg
Cleland *et al.* 1985	Enalapril	40 mg od	36.5 mg
Creager *et al.* 1985	Enalapril	20 mg bd	23.6 mg
Mortality			
CONSENSUS 1986	Enalapril	20 mg bd	18.4 mg
VHeFT II 1991	Enapapril	10 mg bd	15.0 mg
SOLVD (T) 1991	Enalapril	10 mg bd	16.6 mg
SAVE* 1992	Captopril	50 mg tds	NA†

*Post-MI patients.
†79% in captopril group taking 150 mg/day.

Side-effect profile in severe heart failure

Initial experience with ACE inhibitors was with large doses in severely ill patients treated with very high doses of diuretics — exactly the circumstances we now know to carry the greatest risk of adverse events. Despite this, the frequency of serious side-effects in CONSENSUS I was remarkably low.[13]

Even in elderly and severely ill patients, the mean change in blood pressure in the enalapril group was only 10/7 mmHg, compared with 4/2 mmHg in the placebo group. Although baseline creatinine was elevated at 130 μmol/l and the mean daily dose of frusemide was 217 mg, serum creatinine actually fell in 24% of enalapril-treated patients and increased by more than 100% in only 11% of patients.

Side-effect profile in mild-to-moderate heart failure

The side-effect profile in patients with mild-to-moderate heart failure is even more reassuring. Reliable data on this are available from the vast experience in SOLVD.

First-dose hypotension

In SOLVD 7402 outpatients were given an enalapril challenge of 2.5 mg twice daily for 2–7 days.[14] The average first-dose reduction in blood pressure was 6/4 mmHg. Only 2.2% of patients developed symptomatic hypotension, which occurred as infrequently in those with a starting systolic blood pressure below 120 mmHg as it did in those with higher blood pressure. The fall in systolic blood pressure among patients in NYHA class III and IV was significantly greater than those in NYHA class I and II (mean decrease 6.3 versus 5.1 mmHg, P=0.02). Seventy-eight per cent of those who experienced first-dose hypotension were willing to continue in the trial. The average fall in systolic blood pressure in symptomatic patients was 9.7 mmHg, compared with 6.1 mmHg in those who did not report symptoms (P=0.003).

> Among patients in NYHA class III or IV, 78% of those who experienced first-dose hypotension were willing to continue in the trial

Long-term dizziness and hypotension

In the 4-year follow-up of patients in the treatment arm of SOLVD, dizziness and fainting were reported by approximately 50% of placebo-treated patients.[10,15] The excess in the enalapril group was small — 7%. The long-term average reduction in blood pressure with enalapril was only 5/4 mmHg.

Early renal dysfunction

Of 7402 SOLVD outpatients who received an enalapril challenge for 2–7 days, only 0.2% developed significant renal dysfunction.[10, 14] The average increase in creatinine with enalapril was 1.8 μmol. 9.7% of patients had an increase of more than 20% in their pretreatment serum creatinine concentration (mean increase 33 μmol/l). The average increase in blood urea with enalapril was 0.21 mmol/l; 22% of patients had an increased blood urea of more than 20% (mean increase 2.3 mmol/l). Patients in NYHA class III or IV had a greater average increase in blood urea than those in class I or II (0.35 mmol/l versus 0.19 mmol/l).

Long-term renal dysfunction

Over the 4-year follow-up in the treatment arm of SOLVD, mean serum creatinine concentration increased by 8.8 μmol/l in the enalapril group. Long-term significant increases in creatinine (i.e.

concentration >177 µmol/l) occurred in 3% more enalapril-treated than placebo-treated patients.[10, 15]

Early hyperkalaemia

Of the 7402 SOLVD outpatients who received an enalapril challenge for 2–7 days, only 1 developed significant hyperakalaemia.[10,14] The average increase in potassium during this period was 0.1 mmol/l. Six per cent of patients had a greater than 20% increase in serum potassium concentration (mean increase 1.07 mmol/l). Patients in NYHA class III or IV had a significantly greater increase in potassium concentration than those with class I or II heart failure.

> Of the 7402 SOLVD outpatients who received an enalapril challenge for 2–7 days, only 1 developed significant hyperkalaemia

Long-term changes in potassium

Over the 4-year follow-up of the SOLVD treatment arm, the mean serum potassium rose by 0.2 mmol/l in the enalapril group.[10,15] Only 4% more enalapril-treated patients than placebo-treated patients had a significant increase in potassium (i.e. to a concentration >5.5 mmol/l).

Cough

Cough is commonly reported by heart failure patients and was noted in 31% of placebo-treated patients during the 4-year follow-up in the treatment arm of SOLVD.[10,15] Cough has not, however, been a common cause of treatment discontinuation in the large trials. In the treatment arm of SOLVD, only 6% more enalapril-treated patients complained of cough. In VHeFT II, only 1% of patients in each treatment group (H-ISDN and enalapril) were withdrawn from the trial because of cough.

Other adverse effects

Taste disturbance, skin rash, leukopenia and angioedema have rarely been reported in the clinical trials.[10,14,15] Usually, the frequency of these complaints has been no greater with ACE inhibitors than with placebo.

Usually, the frequency of complaints has been no greater with ACE inhibitors than with placebo

Conclusions

The evidence from large placebo-controlled trials is that high doses of ACE inhibitors are remarkably well-tolerated in heart failure, particularly among patients with mild to moderate symptoms. Equally importantly, the trials tell us that many side-effects attributable to ACE inhibitors, such as cough and dizziness, are common in patients with heart failure not receiving such treatment. This means that they should not automatically be blamed on ACE inhibitor therapy if they develop in a patient receiving this treatment. Other explanations, such as pulmonary oedema for cough and arrhythmia for dizziness, must always be considered first (see below).

Many side-effects attributable to ACE inhibitors, such as cough and dizziness, are common in patients with heart failure not receiving such treatment

Cost of treatment

Another concern about ACE inhibitors — their cost — is also unjustified. Heart failure is extremely expensive, accounting for 1.2% of total health care expenditure in many countries. About two-thirds to three-quarters of this outlay is due to the cost of hospitalization.[9] Because hospitalization is so expensive, any therapy that reduces the need for admission and treatment will substantially offset its own costs and the overall cost of heart failure. Indeed, the cost of 1 year of treatment with an ACE inhibitor is roughly similar to the cost of one hospital bed per day. For this reason, ACE inhibitors probably pay for themselves and may even, as suggested in several studies, actually lead to cost savings. Even using the very conservative estimate that 40% of patients might require inpatient initiation of therapy (thus incurring the cost of hospital care), ACE inhibitors are remarkably cost-effective (Table 8.5).[9]

The cost of 1 year of treatment with an ACE inhibitor is roughly similar to the cost of one hospital bed per day

TABLE 8.5 Cost per quality adjusted life for the year 1990.	
ACE inhibitor for mild–moderate CHF*	£502
Pacemaker implant	£1100
Valve replacement for aortic stenosis	£1140
Hip replacement	£1180
CABG (left main stenosis and severe angina)	£2090
Kidney transplant	£4710
Breast cancer screening	£5780
Heart transplant	£7840
CABG (single-vessel disease and moderate angina)	£18830
Hospital haemodialysis	£21970

*Treatment initiated in 40% one-day inpatients and 60% in general practice (i.e. in the community).
CABG, coronary artery bypass grafting.

How to use ACE inhibitors to treat heart failure

Whom to treat

Provided the left ventricular systolic dysfunction has been confirmed, and no major contraindication is present, every patient with heart failure should receive a trial of ACE inhibitor therapy. There are no absolute contraindications to ACE inhibitor treatment, though it should be introduced cautiously, sometimes even under observation in hospital among groups of patients believed to have a higher risk of side-effects (Table 8.6).

Every patient with heart failure due to left ventricular systolic dysfunction should be considered for treatment with an ACE inhibitor

How to treat

Certain precautions should be taken before treatment is started (Fig. 8.9). A small first dose is usually prescribed (for example, captopril 6.25 mg or enalapril 2.5 mg). Treatment can be started at any time of day. It has been common practice to have the patient sit or lie down for 1–2 h after the first dose, or for the dose to be taken after retiring to bed. As long as the patient does not experience significant dizziness or light-headedness after the first dose, regular treatment can be initiated, usually at an intermediate dose such as captopril 12.5 mg three times a day or enalapril 5 mg twice daily. After 3–7 days, the patient should be reviewed to:

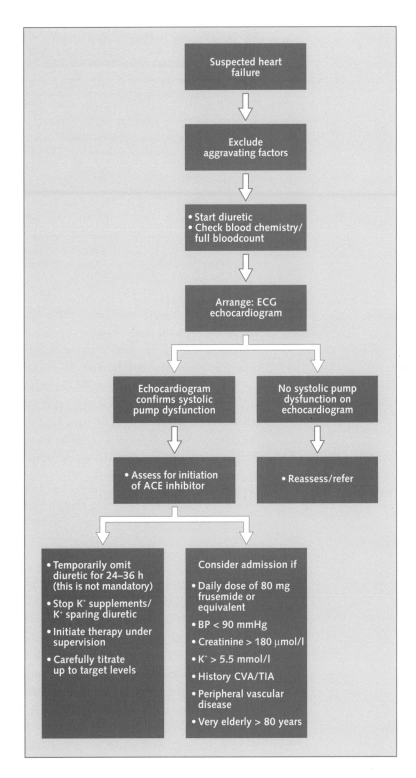

FIG. 8.9 Guidelines for starting ACE inhibitors.

TABLE 8.6 Patients with systolic dysfunction thought to be at increased risk of hypotension/renal dysfunction.

- Severe heart failure (NYHA class IV), frusemide equivalent dose >80 mg
- Low systolic blood pressure (<90 mmHg)
- Low serum sodium (<130 mmol/l)
- Possible hypovolaemia (low jugular venous pressure, recent diuresis/fluid loss, high diuretic dose, combination diuretic therapy)
- Additional vasodilator treatment (excluding nitrates)
- Existing renal dysfunction (creatinine ≥180 μmol/l and/or K$^+$>5.5 mmol/l)
- Peripheral vascular disease
- Very elderly (>80 yrs)

Other patients at increased risk include those with:
- Severe diabetes mellitus with associated vascular and renal disease
- Severe generalized atherosclerosis (especially if intermittent claudication and arterial bruits are present)
- Severe chronic obstructive airways disease and pulmonary heart disease ('cor pulmonale')

- recheck blood chemistry;
- check for *symptomatic* hypotension (hypertension is not a reason to stop close titration or discontinue therapy);
- further titrate the dose of ACE inhibitor.

Provided the patient has not experienced a significant rise in creatinine or potassium (>200 μmol/l or >5.5 mmol/l respectively), the dose of ACE inhibitor should be increased. The target dose is that used in the clinical trials — captopril 50 mg three times a day or enalapril 10 mg twice daily.

> The target dose is that used in the clinical trials — captopril 50 mg three times a day or enalapril 10 mg twice daily

How to deal with side-effects

First-dose hypotension. Some fall in blood pressure is to be expected after ACE inhibitor therapy is initiated but, as pointed out earlier, it is usually small and asymptomatic. Rarely, a patient experiences a large and symptomatic reduction in pressure. If this occurs, it is important to re-evaluate the case:
- has obstructive valve disease been missed?
- does the patient have significant pulmonary disease?
- does the patient have diastolic rather than systolic dysfunction?
- has the patient become volume depleted?

Limiting hypotension is unusual unless the patient has very severe end-stage heart failure. The most common cause of hypotension is sodium and water depletion due to overly vigorous diuresis, and the majority of patients will tolerate a second attempt to reintroduce treatment after a few days of reduced diuretic therapy.

> Some fall in blood pressure is to be expected after ACE inhibitor therapy is initiated, but it is usually small and asymptomatic

Dizziness. Dizziness during longer-term treatment is also usually due to dehydration caused either by diuretics or some other cause of fluid loss such as diarrhoea and vomiting. Patients with syncope should always be investigated for arrhythmia.

Renal dysfunction and hyperkalaemia. Small rises in urea and creatinine are common and of no significance. If serum creatinine rises by more than 25% or reaches more than 200 µmol/l the diuretic dose should be reduced in the absence of signs of fluid retention (oedema or raised jugular venous pressure). If there is fluid retention, the dose of ACE inhibitor should be halved and the patient reassessed within 3–4 days. If the creatinine remains elevated, ACE inhibitor treatment should be stopped and the patient referred for specialist advice. The same approach is appropriate if serum potassium rises above 5.5 mmol/l.

Patients who are well-established on an ACE inhibitor may also experience intermittent increases in urea, creatinine and potassium. These will usually be the result of an intercurrent illness leading to dehydration and should prompt diuretic dose-reduction or withdrawal; if there is a major disturbance of blood chemistry, the ACE inhibitor should also be stopped temporarily. A close watch should be kept on renal function until it returns to normal.

Co-prescription of a non-steroidal anti-inflammatory drug (NSAID) commonly leads to impaired renal function. NSAIDs should not be prescribed for patients with heart failure unless absolutely necessary; advice about over-the-counter NSAIDs should also be given.

Co-prescription of potassium-conserving diuretics and potassium supplements increases the risk of hyperkalaemia and should not be employed unless the serum potassium concentration remains persistently below 3.5 mmol/l.

Cough. As cough may indicate the development of pulmonary oedema, clinical examination supplemented by chest radiography should always be considered. If a very troublesome cough develops, ACE inhibitor therapy may have to be stopped. Alternatively, as recently reported, inhaled sodium cromogylcate may be given. If the ACE inhibitor is stopped, losartan, an angiotensin II receptor antagonist, or H-ISDN, may be appropriate substitutes.

References

1 Dargie HJ, McMurray J. Chronic heart failure: epidemiology, aetiology, pathophysiology and treatment. In: Rowlands DJ ed. *Recent Advances in Cardiology II*. Edinburgh: Churchill Livingstone, 1992; 73–114.

2 Cleland JGF. *The Clinician's Guide to ACE Inhibition*. Edinburgh: Churchill Livingstone, 1993.

3 Schofield PM, Brooks NH, Lawrence GP *et al*. Which vasodilator drug in patients with chronic heart failure? A randomised comparison of captopril and hydralazine *Br J Clin Pharmacol* 1991; **31**: 25–32.

4 Cohn JN, Johnson G, Ziesche S *et al*. A comparison of enalapril with hydrazaline-isosorbide dinitrate in the treatment of chronic congestive heart failure. *N Eng J Med* 1991; **325**: 303–310.

5 Bayliss J, Norell MS, Canepa-Anson R *et al*. Clinical importance of the renin-angiotensin system in chronic heart failure: a double-blind comparison of captopril and prazosin. *Br Med J* 1985; **290**: 1861–1865.

6 The Captopril–Digoxin Multicenter Research Group. Comparative effects of therapy with captopril and digoxin in patients with mild to moderate heart failure. *JAMA* 1988; **259**: 539–544.

7 Kleber FX, Niemiller L, Doering W. Impact of converting enzyme inhibition on progression of chronic heart failure. *Br Heart J* 1992; **67**: 289–296.

8 Pflugfelder PW, Baird MG, Tonkon MJ, Di Bianco R, Pitt B. Clinical consequences of angiotensin-converting enzyme inhibitor withdrawal in chronic heart failure: a double-blind placebo-controlled study of quinapril. *J Am Coll Cardiol* 1993; **22**: 1557–1563.

9 McMurray J, Davie A. The pharmacoeconomics of ACE inhibitors in chronic heart failure. *Pharmacoeconomics* 1996; **9**: 188–197.

10 The SOLVD Investigators. Effect of enalapril on survival in patients with reduced left ventricular ejection fractions and congestive heart failure. *N Engl J Med* 1991; **325**: 293–302.

11 Cohn JN, Archibald DG, Ziesche S *et al*. Effect of vasodilator therapy on mortality in chronic congestive heart failure: results of a Veterans Administration Cooperative Study. *N Engl J Med* 1986; **314**: 1547–1552.

12 CONSENSUS Trial Study Group. Effects of enalapril on mortality in severe congestive heart failure. Results of the cooperative north Scandinavian enalapril survival study. *N Engl J Med* 1987; **316**: 1429–1435.

13 Kjekshus JD, Swedberg K, for the CONSENSUS Trial Study Group. Tolerability of enalapril in congestive heart failure. *Am J Cardiol* 1988; **62**(Supppl. A): 67A–72A.

14 Kostis JB, Shelton BJ, Yusuf S *et al*. Tolerability of enalapril initiation by patients with left ventricular dysfunction: results of the medication challenge phase of the studies of left ventricular dysfunction. *Am Heart J* 1994; **128**: 358–364.

15 Kostis JB, Shelton BJ, Gosselin G *et al*. Adverse effects of enalapril in the Studies of Left Ventricular Dysfunction: SOLVD. *Am Heart J* 1996; **131**: 350–355.

Treatment of Heart Failure: Digoxin

SUMMARY POINTS

- Although digoxin is effective in reducing the heart rate of patients with atrial fibrillation, it is contraindicated in situations of re-entry tachycardia, for example, in Wolff–Parkinson–White syndrome, where the drug can increase the heart rate and cause ventricular fibrillation
- Digoxin has a weak chronic inotropic effect and causes a diuresis
- There are very few data to show whether adding digoxin to current treatment with an angiotensin-converting enzyme inhibitor and diuretic combination confers any advantage
- The issue of whether digoxin causes an increase in mortality in patients with acute myocardial infarction is controversial
- Drug interactions known to occur with digoxin include quinidine, amiodarone and verapamil

Cardiac glycosides and related compounds have been given to patients with heart disease for many centuries. There is mention in the ancient Indian, Egyptian and Roman literature[1] of the use of such substances to treat conditions which might now well be referred to as heart failure. The modern use of cardiac glycosides, digitalis in particular, began with the publication of *An Account of the Foxglove* by William Withering in 1785.[2] This was notable not just because it described the use of an extract from the foxglove, *Digitalis purpurea*, to treat heart failure, but because of the care with which the evidence had been obtained and documented to demonstrate efficacy and to describe the side-effects and method of administration.

Since that time, digitalis (or nowadays, the chemically manufactured compound digoxin) has been widely used to treat patients with various forms of heart failure.[3] However, the use of digoxin in patients with heart failure in sinus rhythm has been controversial almost since the beginning of this century,[4–7] and the debate is not yet over. Several recent withdrawal studies[8–10] have revived enthusiasm for the use of digoxin. The results of the large mortality study called DIG, recently reported from the National Institutes of Health in the USA, has not shown any impact on mortality of digoxin in patients with heart failure.

> Use of digoxin in patients with heart failure in sinus rhythm has been controversial almost since the beginning of this century

Clinical efficacy of digoxin in atrial fibrillation

A crucial distinction must be made between the use of digoxin in patients with atrial fibrillation and those in sinus rhythms. Digoxin undoubtedly reduces the heart rate at rest in patients with fast atrial fibrillation, resulting in substantial benefit in many clinical situations. However, the evidence that digoxin maintains patients in sinus rhythm after cardioversion from atrial fibrillation, or prevents episodes of atrial fibrillation in those with paroxysmal atrial fibrillation, is questionable and doubtful.

Digoxin has been used in patients with nodal tachycardia, but care must be taken to distinguish them from individuals with re-entry tachycardia, for whom digoxin is contraindicated. In the presence of a re-entry pathway in the Wolff–Parkinson–White (WPW) syndrome, digoxin increases the conduction velocity through the additional atrioventricular pathway, such that in the presence of atrial fibrillation the ventricular rate is sufficiently fast to lead to ventricular fibrillation and sudden death.

> Patients with nodal tachycardia must be distinguished from those with re-entry tachycardia, for whom digoxin is contraindicated

Efficacy of digoxin in patients with heart failure in sinus rhythm

A large number of studies have claimed to show that digoxin is of benefit in patients with heart failure in sinus rhythm.[4, 6, 11, 12] Some are old reports that predate the introduction of diuretics for the treatment of heart failure and are not relevant to current medical practice. It may well be that digoxin has a direct diuretic action in the kidney, and other extracardiac actions that benefit patients with heart failure in sinus rhythm in the absence of other modern treatments, but the effect would not be useful today.

That digoxin exerts a chronic inotropic effect is undoubted,[13, 14] though occasionally questioned.[15] It appears to improve the function of the heart and cause diuresis, particularly in patients with initial sodium and water retention.[14] If sodium and water retention is already optimally treated with a diuretic, the evidence for benefit from digoxin is less clear.[15]

In order to clarify the nature of the controversy concerning digoxin, it is necessary to identify the critical clinical questions concerning its use in the context of currently available drugs. The question is not whether digoxin is positively inotropic, either acutely or chronically, in patients with heart failure and in sinus rhythm, nor whether it can be shown to be beneficial for heart failure in selected groups of patients and under particular circumstances. The key question for the clinician is whether a patient who has received optimal treatment with angiotensin-converting enzyme (ACE) inhibitors and a combination of diuretics benefits further from the addition of digoxin.

> The key question is whether a patient who has received optimal treatment with ACE inhibitors and a combination of diuretics benefits further from the addition of digoxin

This issue is crucial because the current initial treatment for overt heart failure is the careful use of an ACE inhibitor combined with a diuretic. In 1982, Lee and colleagues showed that patients with fluid overload and a third heart sound benefited from the use of digoxin.[14] That is to be expected, but exactly the same result might have been obtained by the propitious use of an ACE inhibitor and a diuretic. Indeed, the clinical and haemodynamic benefit[13] is probably related to change in total body weight.[16] There may be subgroups of patients in whom digoxin is particularly useful in addition to ACE inhibitors and diuretics, but they need to be identified in carefully controlled clinical trials.

> Any subgroups of patients in whom digoxin is particularly useful in addition to ACE inhibitors and diuretics need to be identified in carefully controlled clinical trials

Most of the many investigations into the use of digoxin conducted in the last century,[6, 7, 11, 12] have been withdrawal or observational studies. Some included patients in atrial fibrillation. Very few would fulfil current criteria for a proper clinical trial. One meta-analysis[7] and one overview have been published recently.[6] The meta-analysis found seven trials in the world literature which fulfilled the criteria for a modern study, but only

TABLE 9.1 Trials of digoxin in chronic heart failure.

Author	Date	Patients	Exercise capacity	Symptoms or heart failure score
Lee et al.[14]	1982	25		Improved
Fleg et al.[17]	1982	30	Unchanged (−2%)	
Taggart et al.[18]	1983	22		Unchanged
Guyatt et al.[19]	1988	20	Unchanged (+5%)	Variable
German and Austrian Xamoterol Study Group[20]	1988	213	Unchanged (+6%)	Variable
Captopril–Digoxin Multicenter Research Group[21]	1988	196	Unchanged (+10%)	Unchanged

six were included in the overview (Table 9.1).[14, 17–21] The one rejected from the overview was a withdrawal study.[10]

The authors of the meta-analysis concluded that there was evidence that the total number of control patients withdrawn from studies was statistically significantly different from the number of digoxin patients withdrawn (64/354 placebo versus 25/357 digoxin, odds ratio 0.28, 95% confidence interval 0.16–0.49). The overview was unable to show any benefit to patients in terms of symptoms or exercise capacity. The numbers were far too small to show any benefit in terms of mortality.

Thus, two independent reviews, one by an advocate of digoxin and one by a doubter, found the best evidence for the efficacy of digoxin to be based on the number of patients withdrawn from trials rather than a symptomatic end-point such as exercise capacity, shortness of breath or fatigue. Withdrawal from a study is not a secure end-point for the demonstration of efficacy and was not predetermined in the studies. These data do not lie easily with the common claim that digoxin unequivocally decreases symptoms in patients with heart failure.

The best evidence for the efficacy of digoxin is based on the number of patients withdrawn from trials, rather than a symptomatic end-point

Withdrawal studies

Three withdrawal studies have recently been reported (Table 9.2).[9–11] The problem with this approach to evaluating the efficacy of digoxin, or any other drug, is that it does not answer the clinical question of whether adding digoxin to a patient's current treatment confers advantage. It addresses instead the issue of whether the patient who has been started on the drug should have it stopped. The difference is crucial when considering positive inotropic drugs (Table 9.3). For example, it has been claimed that amrinone damages the myocardium, but that deterioration in myocardial function is seen only after the drug is withdrawn.

TABLE 9.2 Recent withdrawal trials with digoxin.
NYHA class II or III, EF <35% on treatment
DiBianco et al.[10] (n=230)
Lower EF on placebo, deaths 3/49 placebo versus 3/62 digoxin Withdrawals: placebo 26/49 digoxin 11/62, $P<0.01$
Packer et al.[8] (n=178)
Lower EF and reduced functional capacity on placebo Withdrawals: placebo 23/93, digoxin 4/85, $P<0.001$
Uretsky et al. (n=88)[9]
Reduced exercise capacity and weight increase on placebo Withdrawals: placebo 21/46 digoxin 10/42, $P<0.04$

NYHA, New York Heart Association; EF, ejection fraction.

TABLE 9.3 Critique of recent withdrawal trials of digoxin.
Wrong clinical question — withdrawal, not initiation
Key clinical question is whether digoxin added to optimal treatment with angiotensin-converting enzyme inhibitors and diuretics is advantageous
These two trials test efficacy of digoxin, *not* a therapeutic strategy
Interpretation of the results is ambiguous; compatible with digoxin being harmful
Withdrawal studies should not be and are not used to test efficacy of drugs

A positive inotropic drug might have two effects, probably with different time-courses. The first might be an advantageous increase in cardiac output consequent upon the positive inotropic action, and the second might be a deleterious potential increase in cell death (Table 9.4). Deterioration in a patient's condition after digoxin withdrawal might therefore lead to two possible conclusions: that digoxin was beneficial because of its positive inotropic effect, or it was doing harm because it damaged the myocardium and the harmful effect only became evident on withdrawal because it was concealed by the positive inotropic action during administration. Thus the trial does not resolve the question of whether the drug is beneficial. Such problems are an unavoidable consequence of withdrawal studies, which are therefore not suitable for demonstrating efficacy when initiating treatment with a new drug

> Digoxin may do good because of its positive inotropic effect, or harm because it damages the myocardium and the damage only becomes evident on withdrawal

TABLE 9.4 Adverse effect of positive inotropic drugs: putative mechanisms.

Increased ischaemia, hibernation or stunning

Worsening heart failure due to excessive workload

'Cardiomyopathy of overload', metabolic exhaustion

Arrhythmias

Apoptosis

Hypotension

This phenomenon is particularly evident in the milrinone–digoxin study.[10] Subjects who increased their exercise tests most were those who remained on digoxin with no alteration to their treatment whatsoever. Patients in whom digoxin was withdrawn had a reduced exercise capacity compared to those who continued on the drug, but did not exhibit a change in exercise capacity during the study. This unexpected result presents very real difficulties in interpretation. It appears that the patients could not have been in a stable condition at randomization.

Drugs in heart failure can be advantageous for three reasons:
- heart failure may be prevented;
- symptoms may be minimized;
- mortality may be reduced.

The evidence that digoxin is beneficial in preventing or treating symptoms is not strong, and other approaches such as ACE inhibitors and combinations of diuretics appear to be preferable. The very few studies that have compared digoxin with ACE inhibitors (Tables 9.5 and 9.6) show no advantage with digoxin.[21–23]

> The very few studies that have compared digoxin with ACE inhibitors show no advantage with digoxin

TABLE 9.5 Comparisons of digoxin with angiotensin-converting enzyme (ACE) inhibitors.

Trial	Date	Type	*n*
Captopril–Digoxin Multicenter Research Group[21]	1988	Parallel group	300
Alicandri et al.[22]	1987	Cross-over	16
Kromer et al.[23]	1990	Cross-over	19

There were no differences between digoxin and ACE inhibitors except that ACE inhibitors increased exercise time more in the study of Alicandri et al.[22]

TABLE 9.6 The captopril–digoxin study.

300 patients, mild-to-moderate heart failure, possible wean off digoxin Randomized to digoxin, captopril or placebo

Digoxin increased left ventricular ejection fraction more than captopril

Compared to placebo

Digoxin did not affect exercise time, NYHA class or VPBs

Captopril increased exercise time, improved NYHA class and reduced VPBs

Digoxin and captopril had fewer hospital admissions or study withdrawals

NYHA, New York Heart Association; VPBs, ventricular premature beats. From the Captopril–Digoxin Multicenter Research Group[21] with permission.

Digoxin and mortality

No mortality studies in heart failure have been conducted using digoxin, yet surrogate end-points such as exercise time and clinical symptoms are unsatisfactory. A large number of positive inotropic drugs have been shown to have harmful effects in heart failure, including increased mortality. The list includes flosequinan, xamoterol, vesarinone, amrinone, milrinone, ibopamine and pimbobendan. The burden of proof of safety lies with those who wish to use positive inotropic drugs in heart failure.

The burden of proof of safety lies with those who wish to use positive inotropic drugs in heart failure

A number of observational studies suggest a possible increase in mortality if digoxin is given in the context of acute myocardial

133

infarction (Table 9.7).[6] The issue has been partly resolved by a large study which was recently reported from the USA. The investigation, called DIG, involved 8000 patients and had mortality as its end-point. About half of the patients are receiving digoxin *de novo* and the other half are involved in a withdrawal trial. The results showed that digoxin conferred no benefit in terms of reducing mortality.

TABLE 9.7 Probability that digoxin is an independent cause of mortality when given to patients in the year following acute myocardial infarction.

Authors	*n*	% on Digoxin	Follow-up months	*P*
Moss *et al.*	812	19	14	<0.01
Ryan *et al.* (CASS)	892	21	55	<0.1
Madsen *et al.*	1300	37	12	<0.1
Bigger *et al.*	504	45	23	<0.1
Byington (BHAT)	1921	13	25	NS
Muller *et al.* (MILIS)	903	31	25	0.14
Digitalis Subcommittee	867	31	31	<0.001

From Poole-Wilson *et al.*[6]

Clinical use of digoxin

The clinical use of digoxin for chronic heart failure can be summarized as follows:
- oral administration at a dose of 0.0625–0.5 mg daily;
- usual maintenance dose 0.25 mg daily;
- initial loading dose of 1.0–1.5 mg in doses of 0.5 mg spread over 24 h can be given, but is not essential unless an early effect is required;
- absorption between 55% and 90%;
- excretion largely through the kidney;
- peak effect between 2 and 6 h;
- half-life approximately 36 h;
- therapeutic concentration is 1–2 ng/ml.

The dose needs to be adjusted in the young and elderly. Older people are particularly sensitive to digoxin. Digoxin can cause arrhythmias, particularly if plasma potassium is low. All patients should have their renal function and plasma potassium measured before digoxin is begun. A simple formula for the adjustment of the dose in the presence of mild renal failure is:
- creatinine clearance 10–25 ml/min: 0.125 mg daily;

- creatinine clearance 26–49 ml/min: 0.125 mg in the morning and 0.0625 mg in the evening;
- creatinine clearance 50–79 ml/min: 0.025 mg daily.

Digoxin should be used with great care in severe renal failure. The dose must be greatly reduced and the serum concentration measured. The serum concentration of digoxin taken at least 6 h after the last dose can be used as a guide to dose, and should be between 1 and 2 ng/ml.

> The serum concentration of digoxin taken at least 6h after the last dose can be used as a guide to dose, and should be between 1 and 2 ng/ml

Drug interactions

Several drugs have been shown to interact with digoxin. The best known is quinidine, which interferes with the excretion, volume of distribution and bioavailability of digoxin. The dose of digoxin should be reduced by 50% and the serum concentration measured. Similar precautions should be taken with amiodarone and verapamil. Caution should always be considered when combining digoxin with antiarrhythmic or positive inotropic drugs. Care is also needed in the presence of myxoedma, hypoxaemia, hypokalaemia and hypomagnesaemia.

> Caution should always be considered when combining digoxin with antiarrhythmic or positive inotropic drugs

Conclusions

Digoxin is useful for controlling the resting heart rate in patients with heart failure and atrial fibrillation, but its benefit is less well-established in patients with heart failure in sinus rhythm. At present, other treatments, such as ACE inhibitors, diuretics and combinations of diuretics, should be considered before the introduction of digoxin. A simple scheme is shown in Table 9.8.[5] Patients most likely to obtain benefit from digoxin are those with moderately severe heart failure who still have unacceptable symptoms after treatment with ACE inhibitors and diuretics.

> Patients most likely to obtain benefit are those with moderately severe heart failure who still have unacceptable symptoms after receiving ACE inhibitors and diuretics

Trials can only be guides to clinical care. Digoxin is an ancient

TABLE 9.8 Digoxin as first drug after diuretic in the treatment of heart failure.	
Indications	Contraindications
Atrial fibrillation	Diastolic heart failure
Supraventricular tachycardia	Mitral stenosis (no atrial fibrillation or RV failure)
Contraindication to ACE inhibitor	Aortic stenosis (no failure)
	Hypertrophic cardiomyopathy
	Mild heart failure (asymptomatic with diuretic and ACE inhibitor)
Unknown	
Severe heart failure	
Mild heart failure	

Adapted from Smith.[5]
ACE, Angiotensin-converting enzyme; RV, right ventricular.

drug and has many friends. Loyalty is an admirable characteristic, but physicians should at least consider the possibility that strongly held opinions may be wrong and exercise caution where the proof of benefit is lacking, at least until further evidence is available.

References

1 Moore DA. William Withering and digitalis. *Br Med J* 1985; **290**: 324.

2 Withering W. *An Account of the Foxglove, and Some of its Medical Uses: with Practical Remarks on Dropsy, and other Diseases.* GJJ and J Robinson, London, 1785.

3 Smith TW. Digoxin in heart failure. *N Engl J Med* 1993; **329**: 51–52.

4 Petch MC. Digoxin for heart failure in sinus rhythm. *Thorax* 1979; **34**: 147–149.

5 Smith TW. Should digoxin be the drug of first choice after diuretics in chronic congestive heart failure? Protagonist's viewpoint. *J Am Coll Cardiol* 1988; **12**: 267–271.

6 Poole-Wilson PA, Robinson K. Digoxin — a redundant drug in the treatment of congestive heart failure. *Cardiovasc Drugs Ther* 1989; **2**: 733–741.

7 Jaeschke R, Oxman AD, Guyatt GH. To what extent do congestive heart failure patients in sinus rhythm benefit from digoxin therapy? A systematic overview and meta-analysis. *Am J Med* 1990; **88**: 279–286.

8 Packer M, Gheorghiade M, Young JB. Randomized, double-blind, placebo-controlled, withdrawal study of digoxin in patients with chronic heart failure treated with converting-enzyme inhibitors. *N Engl J Med* 1993; **329**: 1–7.

9 Uretsky BF, Young JB, Shahidi FE, Yellen LG, Harrison MC, Jolly ML. Randomized study assessing the effect of digoxin withdrawal in patients with mild to moderate chronic congestive heart failure: results of the PROVED trial. *J Am Coll Cardiol* 1993; 22: 955–962.

10 DiBianco R, Shabetai R, Kostuk W, Moran J, Schlant RC, Wright R. A comparison of oral milrinone, digoxin, and their combination in the treatment of patients with chronic heart failure. *N Engl J Med* 1989; **320**: 677–683.

11 Poole-Wilson PA. Digitalis: dead or alive? *Cardiology* 1988; **75** (suppl 1): 103–109.

12 Kulick DL, Rahimtoola SH. Current role of digitalis therapy in patients with congestive heart failure. *JAMA* 1991; **265**: 2995–2997.

13 Arnold SB, Byrd RC, Meister W *et al*. Long-term digitalis therapy improves left ventricular function in heart failure. *N Engl J Med* 1980; **303**: 1443–1448.

14 Lee DC, Johnson RA, Bingham JB *et al*. Heart failure in outpatients: a randomized trial of digoxin versus placebo. *N Engl J Med* 1982; **306**: 699–705.

15 McHaffie D, Purcell H, Mitchell-Heggs P, Guz A. The clinical value of digoxin in patients with heart failure and sinus rhythm. *Q J Med* 1978; **47**: 401–419.

16 Meister W, Arnold SB, Byrd RC, Cheitlin MD, Chatterjee K. Intraindividual discrepancy of the clinical and haemodynamic effects of digoxin. *Eur Heart J* 1983; **4** (suppl E): 109.

17 Fleg JL, Gottlieb SH, Lakatta EG. Is digoxin really important in treatment of compensated heart failure? A placebo-controlled crossover study in patients with sinus rhythm. *Am J Med* 1982; **73**: 244–250.

18 Taggart AJ, Johnston GD, McDevitt DG. Digoxin withdrawal after cardiac failure in patients with sinus rhythm. *J Cardiovasc Pharmacol* 1983; **5**: 229–234.

19 Guyatt GH, Sullivan MJ, Fallen EL *et al*. A controlled trial of digoxin in congestive heart failure. *Am J Cardiol* 1988; **61**: 371–375.

20 The German and Austrian Xamoterol Study Group. Double-blind placebo-controlled comparison of digoxin and xamoterol in chronic heart failure. *Lancet* 1988; **1**: 489–493.

21 The Captopril–Digoxin Multicenter Research Group. Comparative effects of therapy with captopril and digoxin in patients with mild to moderate heart failure. *JAMA* 1988; **259**: 539–544.

22 Alicandri C, Fariello R, Boni E *et al*. Captopril versus digoxin in mild-moderate chronic heart failure: a crossover study. *J Cardiovasc Pharmacol* 1987; **9** (suppl 2): S61–S67.

23 Kromer EP, Elsner D, Riegger AJ. Digoxin, converting-enzyme inhibition (quinalapril), and the combination in patients with congestive heart failure functional class II and sinus rhythm. *J Cardiovasc Pharmacol* 1990; **16**: 9–14.

Other Management Aspects of Heart Failure

SUMMARY POINTS

- The patient and family should receive education and counselling about heart failure syndrome
- Patients should be advised that the doses of their diuretic should be taken to suit their daily schedule
- Patients taking angiotensin-converting enzyme inhibitors should be warned about common side-effects, such as dizziness and cough; a bout of dizziness is often caused by fluid depletion during warm weather or illness
- Non-adherence is a common reason for heart failure hospitalization
- Drugs to avoid in heart failure patients include non-steroidal anti-inflammatory drugs, some calcium channel blockers, tricyclic antidepressants
- Cachexia can be a problem, particularly in elderly patients, and every effort should be taken to ensure that these patients receive adequate nutrition with dietary supplementation if necessary
- Regular activity has manifold benefits and should be encouraged

Education and counselling of the patient and family about heart failure and its treatment are considered to be of great importance. It is also widely believed — though poorly researched — that appropriate attention to lifestyle and other non-pharmacological aspects of the management of heart failure can improve quality of life and help ensure disease stability.

Education about the heart failure syndrome

The patient and family should receive both education and counselling about the heart failure syndrome. To this end, the World Health Organization (WHO)[1] and the US Agency for Health Care Policy and Research (AHCPR)[2] guidelines on heart failure both include booklets aimed at patients and families.[1, 2]

Table 10.1 lists the topics that the AHCPR recommends are covered in discussions.

TABLE 10.1 Suggested topics for patient, family and care-giver education and counselling.

General counselling
Explanation of heart failure and the reason for symptoms
Probable cause of heart failure
Expected symptoms
Symptoms of worsening heart failure
What to do if symptoms worsen
Self-monitoring with daily weights
Explanation of treatment/care plan
Clarification of patient's responsibilities
Importance of cessation of tobacco use
Role of family members or other care-givers in the treatment/care plan
Availability and value of qualified local support group
Importance of obtaining vaccinations against influenza and pneumococcal disease

Prognosis
Life expectancy
Advance directives
Advice for family members in the event of sudden death

Activity recommendations
Recreation, leisure and work activity
Exercise
Sex, sexual difficulties and coping strategies

Dietary recommendations
Sodium restriction
Avoidance of excessive fluid intake
Fluid restriction (if required)
Alcohol restriction

Medications
Effects of medications on quality of life and survival
Dosing
Likely side-effects and what to do if they occur
Coping mechanisms for complicated medical regimens

Importance of compliance with the treatment/care plan

One particularly important aspect of education is to teach the patient to look for early signs of worsening heart failure, and to explain what to do when they occur. The most useful measure patients can take in this regard is to weigh themselves each morning after urinating and before eating. A sustained increase in weight of more than 1.5–2.5 kg (3–5 lb) may indicate increasing fluid retention and the need for treatment modification.

One particularly important aspect of education is to teach the patient to look for early signs of worsening heart failure, and to explain what to do when they occur

Discussion of prognosis

The AHCPR guidelines stress the need to discuss the prognosis with the patient and family.[2] Nevertheless, many doctors do not do this, and even shy away from referring to heart failure at all because patients find it so frightening. However, patients need prognostic information to enable them to make decisions and to plan for the future. Table 10.2 shows average annual mortality rates according to New York Heart Association (NYHA) class.[2] Within each class, mortality is likely to be higher if the patient has severe or progressive symptoms or angina. Conversely, milder symptoms, clinical stability and lack of angina will usually mean a better prognosis.

Patients need prognostic information to enable them to make decisions and to plan for the future

TABLE 10.2 Prognosis in heart failure.

Class of heart failure	Annual mortality rates
NYHA class II	5–10%
NYHA class III	10–20%
NYHA class IV	20–50%

NYHA, New York Heart Association.

Education about heart-failure drug treatments

Diuretics

All diuretics inconvenience patients, who often have to organize their daily activities around the period of most intense diuresis. This can lead to non-adherence and worsening heart failure. Loop diuretics may be preferred by some patients as their effect usually diminishes 4 h after the dose. Patients can be advised that there is no fixed time of day that these drugs need to be taken and that the doses can be timed to suit individual needs. However, if a loop diuretic is taken too late in the day (after 4–6 pm), nocturia may result. If patients need to make a long journey or there is some other reason why a diuresis would be very inconvenient, that day's dose can usually be omitted without any harm.

> If patients need to make a long journey or there is another reason why a diuresis would be very inconvenient, that day's dose can usually be omitted without any harm

Patients who record a sustained increase in weight, or who notice an increase in breathlessness or oedema, may take extra diuretic until their 'dry weight' is restored. Typically, this will mean taking an extra frusemide tablet (40 mg) for 5–7 days. If there is no improvement, medical attention should be sought. Similarly, the patient can be instructed to make downward adjustment of the diuretic dose if there are symptoms of dehydration and hypovolaemia, such as dizziness. This will most commonly be a problem in patients taking an angiotensin-converting enzyme (ACE) inhibitor and is most likely to occur in hot weather or as a result of intercurrent fever, diarrhoea or vomiting.

ACE inhibitors

Patients who are minimally symptomatic, or symptom-free, on diuretics are often puzzled as to why they have been started on an ACE inhibitor. It is important to explain the prophylactic benefits of ACE inhibitors to these patients in order to prevent non-adherence. Advice should also be given about the side-effects of ACE inhibition, most commonly dizziness and cough.[3, 4]

> It is important to explain the prophylactic benefits on ACE inhibitors in order to prevent non-adherence

Dizziness almost always reflects fluid depletion and usually responds to a reduction in diuretic dose. It is most likely to be a problem in warm weather or during an intercurrent pyrexial or fluid-losing illness. If there is severe vomiting or diarrhoea, it is best temporarily to discontinue the ACE inhibitor as well as diuretic.[5] The ACE inhibitor enalapril can itself occasionally cause diarrhoea. Some patients with mild heart failure who feel dizzy on ACE inhibitors even in the absence of hypotension simply cannot tolerate the medication.

Cough in patients with chronic heart failure is often due to pulmonary oedema, and that diagnosis must be excluded before blaming ACE inhibition. Even when it occurs, ACE inhibitor-induced cough in heart failure is rarely severe, and most patients who are informed of the benefits of the treatment choose to continue with it and accept a not too troublesome cough. As the non-angiotensin II-mediated effects of ACE inhibitors are believed to cause the cough, patients who cannot tolerate it may be switched to the angiotensin II receptor antagonist losartan.

> ACE inhibitor-induced cough in heart failure is rarely severe, and most patients who are informed of the benefits of the treatment choose to continue with it

The importance of treatment adherence

Non-adherence (non-compliance) is a problem in many chronic illnesses and may lead to clinical deterioration, hospitalization and death. There is some evidence that this is also the case in heart failure.

Monane *et al.* studied prescription data for elderly patients receiving digoxin for chronic heart failure and found that they were without the drug for an average of 111 out of the 365 days of follow-up.[6] Only 10% of the study group collected enough prescriptions to have medication available daily for the year of follow-up. Ghali *et al.* reported that non-adherence was the commonest reason for heart failure hospitalization; over half of all patients were non-compliant with either pharmacological or dietary recommendations.[7] Vinson *et al.* found that 66 of 140 elderly patients with chronic heart failure were rehospitalized at least once within 6 months of discharge;[8] 38 were readmitted because of recurrent heart failure. Twenty-two of these 38 admissions were felt to have been due to pharmacological or dietary non-compliance and were considered possibly or probably preventable.

> One study reported that non-adherence was the most common reason for heart failure hospitalization

Co-prescribing

Inappropriate co-prescribing is an increasingly common cause of worsening heart failure and hospital readmission.

> Inappropriate co-prescribing is an increasingly common cause of worsening heart failure and hospital readmission

Non-steroidal anti-inflammatory drugs (NSAIDs) cause vasoconstriction, fluid retention and renal dysfunction (particularly renal dysfunction if co-prescribed with an ACE inhibitor). NSAIDs should be prescribed for patients with heart failure only if absolutely necessary. Patients should be warned not to purchase such drugs over the counter.

Calcium channel blockers some agents in this class depress myocardial contractility and should not be prescribed to patients with heart failure unless absolutely necessary. In this context, the safest drugs in the class appear to be amlodipine and verapamil. In one recent large placebo-controlled trial, amlodipine was shown not to aggravate chronic heart failure and even to improve prognosis in patients with chronic heart failure not thought to be due to coronary artery disease.[9]

Depression is common in heart failure. As *tricyclic antidepressant drugs* may further impair cardiac contractility and increase vulnerability to arrhythmias, a selective serotonin reuptake inhibitor may be preferable therapy.

Initiation of conventional doses of *β-blockers* may lead to profound haemodynamic deterioration in patients with heart failure. Though there is interesting new information that β-blockers started at a low dose may be of benefit in at least some types of chronic heart failure, they should only be started under specialist care and careful observation.

Influenza and pneumococcal vaccination

Nichol *et al.* recently reported that in elderly patients, vaccination against influenza leads to an approximately 40% reduction in hospitalizations for CHF.[10]

Pneumococcal vaccination may also be worth considering.

Nutritional and dietary measures

Although much has been written about the supposed importance of dietary measures in the management of heart failure, there is virtually no good evidence of their efficacy from controlled interventions.

Much has been written about the supposed importance of dietary measures, but there is virtually no good evidence of their efficacy

Calorie intake and body weight

Many patients with milder degrees of heart failure are overweight, although cachexia is a feature of advanced disease. Incidentally, obesity itself is a common cause of dyspnoea and of patients being misdiagnosed as having heart failure.

Obesity should be strongly discouraged, as excess body weight increases cardiac work during exercise. Conversely, undernutrition may contribute to the cachexia of severe heart failure. Cardiac cachexia has been found in 35–53% of patients with chronic heart failure. In a recent prospective study of elderly patients in Stockholm, chronic heart failure was the most common single diagnosis in malnourished patients.[11] Both malnutrition and chronic heart failure were independent predictors of mortality at 9 months by multivariate analysis. Muscle wasting in cardiac cachexia also exacerbates exercise intolerance and enhances the sense of fatigue and dyspnoea. Every effort should therefore be made to ensure adequate nutrition in these patients.

Alcohol may contribute to excessive calorie intake as well as having other harmful effects in heart failure. Drug therapy, hepatic and intestinal congestion, malabsorption and electrolyte disorders may all contribute to cachexia.

> Drug therapy, hepatic and intestinal congestion, malabsorption and electrolyte disorders may all contribute to cachexia

Some drugs, notably digoxin, cause anorexia and nausea. Patients frequently complain of similar symptoms when asked to take a large number of tablets at mealtimes. It is worth trying to distribute treatments (particularly once-daily preparations such as digoxin, warfarin and aspirin) over the 24 h rather than administering them all with breakfast. Hyponatraemia often causes anorexia, and electrolyte disturbance should be checked for in the anorexic patient. Similarly, diuretic dosage should be adjusted as required to avoid fluid overload and reduce intestinal and hepatic congestion. Dietary supplementation with protein- and carbohydrate-rich drinks may be of value; for example, Ensure liquid provides 500 kcal as 14% protein, 32% fat and 54% carbohydrate per 500 ml, in addition to minerals and vitamins.

Sodium intake

Although much is made of sodium restriction in chronic heart failure, particularly by authors of American textbooks and guidelines, it is probably not strictly necessary as powerful modern diuretics can usually relieve sodium and water retention.[2] However, unnecessarily large doses of diuretic, or complicated diuretic regimens, many increase the frequency of adverse events such as gout, may exacerbate potassium and magnesium wasting, and may lead to non-compliance.

> Unnecessarily large doses of diuretic, or complicated regimens, may increase the frequency of adverse events, may exacerbate potassium and magnesium wasting, and may lead to non-compliance

Some limitation of sodium intake is, therefore, probably advisable. Unfortunately, however, most dietary sodium is obtained from processed foods rather than adding during cooking or at the table. An added problem is that low-sodium products are expensive. A good rule of thumb is to avoid adding salt while cooking or at the table. If possible, foods with a high sodium content (Table 10.3) should also be avoided. Salt substitutes are available for patients who cannot acquire a taste for unsalted food.

Fat- and water-soluble vitamins

Because fat-soluble vitamin absorption may be diminished in the presence of hepatic and intestinal congestion, supplementation should be considered in cachectic patients.

Although water-soluble vitamins may be lost in association with diuresis, this has not generally been thought to lead to nutritional problems. There are, however, several recent reports concerning diuretic-induced thiamine (vitamin B_1) deficiency, a condition known to cause a form of heart failure (beriberi).[12,13,14] Seligmann et al. reported subclinical thiamine deficiency in patients on long-term treatment with frusemide.[12] The same authors subsequently reported that thiamine supplementation significantly improved left ventricular ejection fraction in these patients.[11]

> Although water-soluble vitamins may be lost in association with diuresis, this has not generally been thought to lead to nutritional problems

TABLE 10.3 Foods which contain a high sodium content.
Bacon, ham, tinned meat, e.g. corned beef, spam, chopped ham and pork
Tinned fish, e.g. salmon, tuna, sardines
Smoked fish, e.g. smoked haddock, kippers
Shellfish
Sausages, made-up meat dishes, e.g. beefburgers, pies
Meat paste and fish paste
Cheese
Pickles, Bovril, Oxo, Marmite, Bisto, gravy browning
Tinned soup, tinned vegetables, tomato juice
Crisps, salted peanuts or any other savoury snacks, peanut butter, milk and white chocolate

Alcohol

Alcohol abuse is a recognized cause of dilated cardiomyopathy. In patients with alcoholic cardiomyopathy, cessation of alcohol intake often results in recovery of ventricular function (Fig. 10.1)[15] and resolution of the symptoms and signs of heart failure. Prognosis is poorest in patients who continue to drink.

It is much more difficult to know what to advise patients with heart failure of another aetiology. Alcohol depresses myocardial contractility, induces atrial fibrillation and may increase vulnerability to ventricular arrhythmias. It is also toxic to skeletal muscle and, if taken as beer, can represent a substantial volume load. For all of these reasons, patients with heart failure are best advised to abstain from alcohol or at least minimize their consumption.

Patients with heart failure are best advised to abstain from alcohol or at least minimize their consumption

Smoking

Smoking has many deleterious effects on the cardiovascular and respiratory systems and is associated with cancers elsewhere. For all these reasons, it should be avoided. Smoking also causes peripheral vasoconstriction in heart failure.[16]

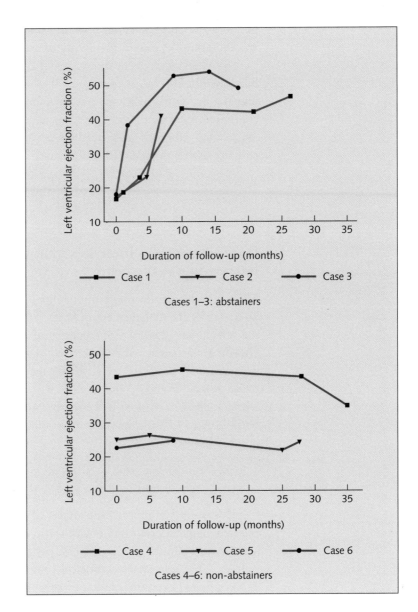

FIG. 10.1 Left ventricular function in abstainers and non-abstainers. (From Jacob et al. 1991.[15])

Activity, sex and work

One of the most important changes in the non-pharmacological management of heart failure has been the recognition of the importance of regular activity for most compensated patients.[17]

Recent studies have shown that patients with compensated heart failure can exercise safely and that regular dynamic exercise:

- improves well-being;
- reduces sympathetic nervous system activity;

147

- improves muscle blood flow and function;
- increases the electrical stability of the heart.

Activities such as walking, cycling, swimming, golfing and bowling should be encouraged. If the patient can physically manage to work without undue symptoms, this too can be continued. In severe heart failure, sexual difficulties are common and sexual practices may need to be modified to accommodate patients with impaired effort tolerance.

> Activities such as walking, cycling, swimming, golfing and bowling should be encouraged

Does educational, lifestyle and non-pharmacological intervention really help?

Three studies suggest that real benefits may accrue from a holistic approach to the management of heart failure. Rosenberg evaluated the effect on dietary adherence and readmission rates of a coordinated team approach to planning, education and supervision.[18] Patient-directed group meetings were central to the programme. Dietary compliance was improved and hospital admissions were reduced to 12% from 46% the previous year, and from 31% to 17% compared with a control group of patients from another hospital.

> Real benefits may accrue from a holistic approach to the management of heart failure

Kostis *et al.* compared the effects of a multi-intervention non-pharmacological programme with those of digoxin and placebo in a three-way parallel group study in patients with congestive heart failure.[19] The non-pharmacological programme included:

1 graduated exercise training three to five times weekly;
2 structured cognitive therapy and stress management;
3 dietary intervention aimed at salt restriction and weight reduction.

The non-pharmacological programme resulted in a significantly greater improvement in exercise tolerance and a significantly greater reduction in scores for anxiety and depression; weight loss was also greater.

Finally, Goodyer and Miskelly reported the impact of medication counselling in a randomized controlled trial involving 100 elderly patients with heart failure.[20] Compliance (measured by tablet count) increased from 61% to 93% in the counselled group. Six-minute walking distance, and distance walked to breathlessness, were significantly better in the counselled group over a 12-week period.

> Six-minute walking distance, and distance walked to breathlessness, were significantly better in the counselled group over a 12-week period

References

1 McMurray J, Gyarfas I, Wenger NK *et al.* Concise guide to the management of heart failure. *Am J Geriatr Cardiol* 1996; **5**: 13–30.

2 Konstam M, Dracup K, Baker D *et al. Heart Failure: Evaluation and Care of Patients with Left-Ventricular Systolic Dysfunction. Clinical Practice Guidelines No. 11.* AHCPR Publication No. 94-0612. Rockville, MD: US Department of Health and Human Services 1994.

3 Kostis JB, Shelton BJ, Yusuf S *et al.* Tolerability of enalapril initiation by patients with left ventricular dysfunction: results of the medication challenge phase of the studies of left ventricular dysfunction. *Am Heart J* 1994; **128**: 358–364.

4 Kostis JB, Shelton B, Gosselin G *et al.* Adverse effects of enalapril in the Studies of Left Ventricular Dysfunction (SOLVD). *Am Heart J* 1996; **131**: 350–355.

5 McMurray J, Matthews DM. Effect of diarrhoea on a patient taking captopril. *Lancet* 1985; **1**: 581.

6 Monane M, Bohn RL, Gurwitz JH, Glynn RJ, Avorn J. Noncompliance with congestive heart failure therapy in the elderly. *Arch Intern Med* 1994; **154**: 433–437.

7 Ghali JK, Kadakia S, Cooper R, Ferlinz J. Precipitating factors leading to decompensation of heart failure. Traits among urban blacks. *Arch Intern Med* 1988; **148**: 2013–2016.

8 Vinson JM, Rich MW, Sperry JC, Shah AS, McNamara T. Early readmission of elderly patients with congestive heart failure. *J Am Geriatr Soc* 1990; **38**: 1290–1295.

9 Elkayam U, Amin J, Mehra A, Vasquez J, Weber L, Rahimtoola SH. A prospective randomized, double-blind, crossover study to compare the efficacy and safety of chronic nifedipine therapy with that of isosorbide dinitrate and their combination in the treatment of chronic congestive heart failure. *Circulation* 1990; **82**: 1954–1961.

10 Nichol KL, Margolis KL, Wuorenma J, Von Sternberg T. The efficacy and cost effectiveness of vaccination against influenza among elderly persons living in the community. *New Engl J Med* 1994; **331**: 778–784.

11 Broqvist M, Arnqvist H, Dahlstrom U, Larsson J, Nylander E, Permert J. Nutritional assessment and muscle energy metabolism in severe chronic congestive heart failure: effects of long-term dietary supplementation. *Eur Heart J* 1994; **15**: 1641–1650.

12 Seligmann H, Halkin H, Rauchfleisch S *et al.* Thiamine deficiency in patients with congestive heart failure receiving long-term furosemide therapy: a pilot study. *Am J Med* 1991; **91**: 151–155.

13 Shimon I, Almog S, Vered Z *et al.* Improved left ventricular function after thiamine supplementation in patients with congestive heart failure receiving long-term furosemide therapy. *Am J Med* 1995; **98**: 485–490.

14 Leslie D, Gheorghiade M. Is there a role for thiamine supplementation in the manage.ment of heart failure? *Am Heart J* 1996; **131**: 1248–1250.

15 Jacob AJ, McLaren KM, Boon NA. Effects of abstinence on alcoholic heart muscle disease. *Am J Cardiol* 1991; **68**: 805–807.

16 Nicolozakes AW, Binkley PF, Leier CV. Hemodynamic effects of smoking in congestive heart failure. *Am J Med Sci* 1988; **296**: 377–380.

17 McKelvie RS, Teo KK, McCartney N, Humen D, Montague T, Yusuf S. Effects of exercise training in patients with congestive heart failure: a critical review. *J Am Coll Cardiol* 1995; **25**: 789–796.

18 Rosenberg S. Patient education leads to better care for heart patients. *HSMHA Health Rep* 1971; **86**: 793–802.

19 Kostis JB, Rosen RC, Cosgrove NM, Shindler DM, Wilson AC. Nonpharmacologic therapy improves functional and emotional status in congestive heart failure. *Chest* 1994; **106**: 996–1001.

20 Goodyer L, Miskelly F, Milligan P. Does encouraging good compliance improve patients' clinical condition in heart failure? *Br J Clin Pract* 1995; **49**: 173–176.

Management of Concomitant Cardiac Problems in Patients with Heart Failure

SUMMARY POINTS

- Concomitant problems found in patients with heart failure are either due to the underlying cause of the disease or are a consequence of it
- Atrial fibrillation is found in a significant proportion of heart failure patients and is associated with a worse prognosis
- Atrial fibrillation in the heart failure patient may be linked to mitral valve disease, thyrotoxicosis or sick sinus syndrome and the restoration of the sinus rhythm is preferred
- Many patients with heart failure have concomitant angina which may be treated medically or surgically
- Amiodarone is the only safe antiarrhythmic to use in chronic heart failure and this should only be given to patients with symptomatic arrhythmias

Many patients with heart failure have concomitant problems that either reflect the underlying cause of their disease (for example, angina reflecting underlying coronary artery disease) or are a consequence of it (for example, ventricular arrhythmias). The management of these concomitant problems is often very different from that in the patient who does not have heart failure.

Atrial fibrillation

Prevalence

Atrial fibrillation is commonly found in patients with heart failure, and the prevalence increases with severity. For example, approximately 50% of patients in the CONSENSUS I trial had atrial fibrillation,[1] compared with only about 10% of those in the treatment arm of SOLVD.[2]

Atrial fibrillation is commonly found in patients with heart failure, and the prevalence increases with severity

Importance

Loss of atrial transport can have very serious consequences in a patient with heart failure due to impaired ventricular function. In these patients, atrial transport may contribute as much as 30% of total cardiac output, and loss of sinus rhythm may herald a significant worsening of the heart failure state. If the ventricular response to atrial fibrillation is very rapid, acute decompensation may occur.

Atrial fibrillation also predisposes to thromboembolism and the risk is greatest in patients who have underlying structural heart disease such as left ventricular (LV) dysfunction. Both clinical and subclinical cerebral embolism are common. For these and perhaps other reasons, atrial fibrillation seems to be associated with a worse prognosis in chronic heart failure (CHF), at least in some studies (Fig. 11.1).[3]

Atrial fibrillation seems to be associated with a worse prognosis in chronic heart failure

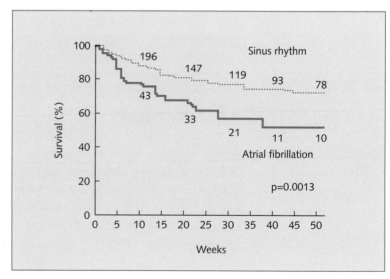

FIG. 11.1 Plots of actuarial one year total survival in patients with sinus rhythm (n=315, broken line) compared with those with atrial fibrillation (n=75, solid line). Numbers along each curve present number of patients at risk. By the Breslow test, survival in atrial fibrillation patients was significantly worse than in sinus rhythm patients (52% versus 71%, P=0.0013). SEM for sinus rhythm and atrial fibrillation patients' survival, respectively, at 25 weeks is ±3% and ±8% and at 50 weeks is ±5% and ±9%

Special issues in heart failure

Four questions should always be asked when a patient presents with heart failure and atrial fibrillation.

Is it the cause or consequence of heart failure?

Atrial fibrillation can precipitate heart failure in a patient without LV systolic dysfunction or valve disease, particularly if the ventricular rate is excessive or if the patient has LV hypertrophy. There is also some evidence that atrial fibrillation may cause a form of cardiomyopathy analogous to tachycardia-induced heart failure in experimental models. In addition, atrial fibrillation is also commonly associated with alcohol abuse. These possibilities should always be considered before assuming atrial fibrillation is a secondary consequence of heart failure.

Could the patient have mitral valve disease?

Mitral valve disease, particularly mitral stenosis, should always be sought in the patient presenting with atrial fibrillation and heart failure, because surgery or balloon valvotomy (for mitral stenosis) may be indicated. Echocardiography is, therefore, mandatory.

Could the patient have thyrotoxicosis?

Thyrotoxicosis (including triiodothyronine (T3) toxicosis) may cause atrial fibrillation and heart failure. Restoration of the euthyroid state is curative.

Could atrial fibrillation be part of the sick sinus syndrome?

Elderly patients with atrial fibrillation may have sick sinus syndrome. This is important for two reasons. First, the symptoms may in part be due to periods of excessive bradycardia; ambulatory electrocardiogram monitoring would help detect them and determine whether pacemaker implantation is indicated. Second, digoxin tends to exacerbate any tendency to bradycardia in these patients; not uncommonly, there may be a need to administer digoxin to control tachycardia and implant a pacemaker to prevent excessive bradycardia. Atrial and dual chamber pacing have particular roles to play. Amiodarone and verapamil may also exacerbate or unmask sick sinus syndrome, particularly if combined with digoxin (N.B. pharmacokinetic interaction).

Vigilance must be maintained during follow-up of patients with CHF receiving rate-limiting treatment for atrial fibrillation. It is not uncommon for sick sinus syndrome to become apparent months or even years after the initial recognition and treatment of atrial fibrillation. This possibility should always be considered if symptomatic or haemodynamic deterioration occurs in patients of this type.

> It is not uncommon for sick sinus syndrome to become apparent months or even years after the initial recognition and treatment of atrial fibrillation

Treatment

Restoration of sinus rhythm

For the reasons outlined above, the optimum treatment for atrial fibrillation in the patient with CHF is restoration of sinus rhythm. This is usually relatively easy in cases with recent-onset atrial fibrillation, particularly if it has occurred in the context of an acute exacerbation of CHF. It is probably best to optimize antifailure therapy, cardiac function and electrolyte balance before attempting electrical cardioversion. For example, congestion should be relieved, mitral and tricuspid regurgitation minimized, LV and left atrial size reduced and sodium, potassium and magnesium concentrations normalized. After about 1 month of treatment with warfarin, cardioversion can be carried out electively. Atrial mechanical function may take several weeks to recover after successful cardioversion and, for that reason, warfarin must be maintained.

> Optimum treatment for atrial fibrillation in the patient with CHF is restoration of sinus rhythm

If cardioversion fails or there is an early relapse back into atrial fibrillation, it is necessary either to accept permanent atrial fibrillation or use amiodarone therapy (p. 160) to enhance the chances of regaining or maintaining sinus rhythm. This choice is easy in the patient who, when restored to sinus rhythm, was clearly symptomatically and clinically improved, but is more difficult in others. However, the benefit of sinus rhythm probably outweighs the cost of long-term, low-dose amiodarone therapy.

Management of the patient with apparently chronic atrial fibrillation is also difficult. If he or she does not have a greatly enlarged left atrium, it is still worth trying to restore sinus rhythm because long-term success (often with amiodarone) is still relatively frequent.

The patient with clear left atrial enlargement has the least chance of restoration of sinus rhythm, though there are still individuals who are surprisingly easy to convert to and maintain in sinus rhythm. Patients may be told about:

- the benefits of regaining sinus rhythm;
- the approach required to try and restore sinus rhythm (i.e. electrical cardioversion and amiodarone);
- the very small hazard associated with this approach;
- the relatively low chance of success.

If the patient wishes to pursue the possibility of restoring sinus rhythm, electrical cardioversion is usually attempted at least once (once not on amiodarone and, if unsuccessful, once after a period of amiodarone treatment or, even, initially after amiodarone treatment).

Control of the ventricular rate

Digoxin is the drug of choice to control the ventricular rate in CHF. Depending on age, weight, renal function and concomitant therapy, a loading dose of 0.375–0.75 mg may be given in three or four divided portions over 24 h. If a loading dose is omitted, a daily maintenance dose will not give steady-state plasma concentrations for at least 7 days and, possibly, for up to 3 weeks if there is marked renal dysfunction. The generally accepted therapeutic plasma concentration range is 0.9–3.2 nmol/l (0.7–2.5 mg/ml). Levels below 0.9 nmol/l are almost always subtherapeutic. Toxicity may be present at any level above this, but is increasingly likely above 3.2 nmol/l. Interestingly, in the large clinical trials of digoxin in CHF, the average daily maintenance dose required to achieve a therapeutic plasma concentration was typically 0.375 mg — much higher than used in ordinary practice.[4]

> In the large clinical trials of digoxin in CHF, the average daily maintenance dose required to achieve a therapeutic plasma concentration was typically 0.375 mg — much higher than used in ordinary practice

In the rare patient who does not respond to an adequate dose of digoxin, every effort should be made to optimize other antifailure therapy and electrolyte balance. Some alternative or additional form of rate-control therapy is also usually required. In practice, this means adding amiodarone, as no other antiarrhythmic agent is suitable or safe (p. 160). Amiodarone, however, increases both the plasma digoxin concentration and warfarin effect by a pharmacokinetic interaction.

It is important not to forget potential thyrotoxicosis in a patient with resistant atrial fibrillation, especially if amiodarone is to be given.

> It is important not to forget potential thyrotoxicosis in a patient with resistant atrial fibrillation

Angina

Coronary artery disease is the commonest cause of heart failure. It is not, therefore, surprising that many patients have concomitant angina. Indeed, the frequency with which these two conditions coexist has been underestimated in the past. The SOLVD registry is probably the most representative population of heart failure patients described in the medical literature.[5] Approximately 60% of the 6273 patients in the registry had a history of angina (and almost 64% had a history of myocardial infarction). Interventional treatment of angina may be medical or surgical. Medical management of angina in patients with heart failure has, until recently, been a particular problem, and the role of surgery has been understated. The place of angioplasty has yet to be properly determined.

> Medical management of angina in patients with heart failure has, until recently, been a particular problem, and the role of surgery has been understated

Medical management

The non-specialist can easily be confused about the value or otherwise of conventional vasodilators in heart failure. Drugs such as nitrates and calcium channel blockers have no role in the treatment of heart failure *per se*. They have not been shown to improve symptoms, exercise tolerance or survival injury. Therefore, their only potential role is in the treatment of concomitant angina.

Until recently, nitrates were the mainstay of antiangina therapy in heart failure. Calcium channel blockers were often used, despite being known to have a detrimental effect on LV function and the heart failure state. β-Blockers were also considered to be contraindicated because of their negative inotropic effect.

Nitrates

Though undoubtedly effective antianginal drugs, nitrates have the major limitation of inducing tolerance if given continuously. Asymmetrical dosing, i.e. leaving a nitrate-free interval, avoids this problem, but at the expense of denying the patient 24-h anti-ischaemic control. In other words, a nitrate-free interval is also a period without anti-ischaemic protection.

Calcium channel blockers

Nifedipine and other short-acting dihydropyridine calcium channel blockers have been shown to worsen heart failure and should not be used in patients with poor LV function.[6] The same is true for diltiazem, which has been shown to increase the risk of patients with impaired LV function developing overt heart failure.[6] The position is less certain with regard to verapamil, which has been given in large trials to patients with heart failure after myocardial infarction without any apparent worsening in prognosis. These patients did not, however, seem to get the benefit from verapamil observed in patients without heart failure.

The real breakthrough in this area came with the introduction of the long-acting dihydropyridine, amlodipine. In a small trial, this drug was shown to improve exercise capacity and suppress the sympathetic nervous system in patients with heart failure treated with full conventional therapy, including, in most cases, an angiotensin-converting enzyme (ACE) inhibitor.[7] Subsequently, in the large Prospective Randomised Amlodipine Survival Evaluation (PRAISE) trial, amlodipine was found to be well-tolerated and safe in patients with severe heart failure.[8] Overall, amlodipine had a neutral effect on mortality; however, somewhat paradoxically, it improved survival in patients with heart failure that was not obviously ischaemic in aetiology.

These new data convincingly show that amlodipine can be used safely in heart failure — not to improve the heart failure state but to treat angina.

Amlodipine can be used safely in heart failure — not to improve the heart failure state but to treat angina

β-Blockers

These may turn out to be the anti-ischaemic treatment of choice in CHF. There is increasing evidence that they may improve the heart failure state *per se* (which neither nitrates nor amlodipine appear to do).[9] β-Blockers are already a proven antianginal treatment and this possible dual mode of action may make them the ideal treatment for a patient with concomitant angina and heart failure. Whether this is ultimately the case will depend on the results of ongoing clinical trials, which should report in the next 5 years.

β-Blockers may turn out to be the anti-ischaemic treatment of choice in CHF

Surgical management

One of the most poorly understood, and paradoxical, findings of the large trials of bypass surgery was that patients with poor LV function had the greatest absolute survival gain from surgery.[10, 11] As the technique of cardiopulmonary bypass has improved, it has become possible to operate safely even on patients with severely depressed LV function. It has also become apparent that, in at least a proportion of cases, LV dysfunction may be, to some degree, reversible. It seems that in these patients, chronic myocardial ischaemia leads to impaired contractility which improves on restoration of an adequate coronary blood flow (so-called hibernating myocardium).

As the technique of cardiopulmonary bypass has improved, it has become possible to operate safely even on patients with severely depressed LV function

Renewed interest in surgical revascularization for patients with heart failure and myocardial ischaemia suggests that, as a rule of thumb, it is advisable to refer any patient with angina, no matter how mild, for further cardiological assessment if that individual is otherwise fit enough (no major concomitant pathology), young enough (generally under 75 years of age) and willing to consider bypass surgery.

Ventricular arrhythmias

No other chronic condition is as arrhythmogenic as heart failure. Up to half of all patients with CHF have non-sustained ventricular tachycardia on ambulatory electrocardiogram monitoring, and about half die a sudden, presumed arrhythmic, death.

> No other chronic condition is as arrhythmogenic as heart failure

Routine antiarrhythmic prophylaxis?

Several large trials of antiarrhythmic prophylaxis are pertinent to CHF. The first and second Cardiac Arrhythmia Suppression Trial (CAST) studies examined the role of class I antiarrhythmic drugs, such as flecainide, in preventing death in patients with impaired LV function and minor ventricular arrhythmias following myocardial infarction.[12] Class I antiarrhythmic agents actually decreased survival in these patients. More recently, two large trials have investigated the role of amiodarone in CHF. In one South American study, Grupo de Estudio de la Sobrevida en la Insuficiencia Cardiaca en Argentina (GESICA), low-dose amiodarone significantly reduced all-cause mortality in patients with severe CHF.[13] However, in a US study, Survival Trial of Antiarrhythmic Therapy in Congestive Heart Failure (CHF-STAT), amiodarone had a neutral effect on mortality.[14]

Further studies with amiodarone are ongoing or planned. For the moment, the main conclusions to be drawn from the available evidence are first, that class I antiarrhythmic drugs are hazardous in CHF, and second, that the only safe antiarrhythmic to use in CHF is amiodarone, although this should not be given prophylactically to asymptomatic patients but should be reserved for patients with symptomatic arrhythmias.

Treatment of asymptomatic arrhythmias

Patients with symptomatic arrhythmias need treatment, but their identification requires a high index of suspicion. Palpitations, dizziness and, particularly, black-outs should alert the doctor to the possibility of a potentially life-threatening arrhythmia. Such patients should be referred *urgently* for further investigation.

> Palpitations, dizziness and, particularly, black-outs should alert the doctor to the possibility of a potentially life-threatening arrhythmia

Management includes investigation by ambulatory electrocardiogram monitoring, exercise testing and, occasionally, sophisticated intracardiac electrophysiological testing. Correctable precipitating or aggravating factors should be excluded (Table 11.1).

If treatment is needed, this will usually be amiodarone. Although there is growing interest in the use of implantable cardioverter defibrillator devices, their precise role in patients with CHF is not clear.

TABLE 11.1 Correctable/precipitating factors for ventricular arrhythmias in CHF.

- Electrolyte disturbance (hypokalaemia, hypomagnesaemia, hyperkalaemia)
- Digoxin toxicity
- Drugs exacerbating pump dysfunction (e.g. calcium channel blockers)
- Drugs causing electrical instability (e.g. anti-arrhythmics, anti-depressants)
- Recurrent myocardial ischaemia

Amiodarone

Properties and use. Amiodarone is a class III antiarrhythmic agent with little or no negative inotropic effect — an almost unique property in this group of drugs. Amiodarone also exhibits the following:[14]

- class I activity;
- blocking of β-adrenoceptors;
- peripheral vasodilator effects;
- antianginal properties.

Amiodarone is slowly absorbed from the gastrointestinal tract and has a very long elimination half-life. A large loading dose (1200–1600 mg for 1–2 weeks) can be used to achieve the full steady-state drug effect as quickly as possible. The dose can then be reduced to 600–800 mg/day for a further 1–3 weeks. It is the author's policy to use 200 mg/day maintenance therapy, although a higher dose is occasionally necessary. Amiodarone is extremely effective in abolishing or controlling both supraventricular (for example, atrial fibrillation) and ventricular tachyarrhythmias.

> Amiodarone is extremely effective in abolishing or controlling both supraventricular (for example, atrial fibrillation) and ventricular tachyarrhythmias

Adverse effects. Apart from general concern about the long-term efficacy of anti-arrhythmic agents, particular attention has been given to the specific adverse events associated with amiodarone. The most common side-effect reported is nausea; the most serious is pneumonitis. Skin pigmentation and disturbance of liver enzymes are not uncommon, and both hypothyroidism and hyperthyroidism may occur. The diagnosis of hyperthyroidism is difficult and should not be based on serum thyroxine (T_4) level alone. Symptoms of weight loss or recurrence of arrhythmias are important pointers. A high serum (T_3) and flat T_4-releasing hormone test are also useful. Regular ophthalmic monitoring is recommended. Photosensitivity can be countered with a high-ultraviolet B sun protection factor sunscreen.

Most of these complications regress over weeks to months following drug withdrawal (although pneumonitis may require steroid treatment and can progress to pulmonary fibrosis). Chest radiographs, thyroid function tests, liver function tests and pulmonary function tests should be monitored serially. Peripheral neuropathy and myopathy have been reported.

Drug interactions. Amiodarone may exert a proarrhythmic effect, particularly if administered with other drugs that prolong the Q-T interval, such as:
- class IA antiarrhythmics (which, in any case, should be avoided in CHF);
- tricyclic antidepressants;
- phenothiazines;
- erythromycin;
- diuretics (causing electrolyte disturbances).

> Amiodarone may exert a proarrhythmic effect, particularly if administered with other drugs that prolong the Q-T interval

Amiodarone increases the effect of warfarin and the concentration of plasma digoxin (the doses of which should be reduced by approximately one-third and one-half, respectively). Amiodarone also interacts with drugs contraindicated in CHF, such as sotalol and calcium antagonists.

References

1 The CONSENSUS Trial Study Group. Effects of enalapril on mortality in severe congestive heart failure. *N Engl J Med* 1987; **316**: 1429–1435.

2 The SOLVD Investigators. Effects of enalapril on survival in patients with reduced left ventricular ejection fractions and congestive heart failure. *N Engl J Med* 1991; **325**: 293–302.

3 Middlekauff HR, Stevenson WG, Stevenson LW. Outcome for advanced heart failure patients with atrial fibrillation. *Cardiol Board Rev* 1992; **9**: 101–102, 107–110.

4 Lancet Editorial. Digoxin: new answers, new questions. *Lancet* 1989; **ii**: 79–80.

5 Bangdiwala SI, Weiner DH, Bourassa MG *et al.* Studies of Left Ventricular Dysfunction (SOLVD) registry: rationale, design, methods and description of baseline characteristics. *Am J Cardiol* 1992; **70**: 347–353.

6 Lancet Editorial. Calcium antagonist caution. *Lancet* 1991; **i**: 885–886.

7 Packer M, Nichol P, Khandheria BR *et al.* Randomized, multicenter, doubleblind, placebo controlled evaluation of amlodipine in patients with mild to moderate heart failure. *J Am Coll Cardiol* 1991; **17**: 24A. (Abstract.)

8 Packer M, O'Connor CM, Ghali JK *et al.* Effect of amlodipine on morbidity and mortality in severe chronic heart failure. *N Engl J Med* 1996; **335**: 1107–1114.

9 Willerson JT. Effect of carvedilol on mortality and morbidity in patients with chronic heart failure. *Circulation* 1996; **94**: 592.

10 Bounous EP, Mark DB, Pollock BG *et al.* Surgical survival benefits for coronary disease patients with left ventricular dysfunction. *Circulation* 1988; **78**(Suppl.): 1151–1157.

11 Yusuf S, Zucker D, Peduzzi P *et al.* Effect of coronary artery bypass graft surgery on survival: overview of 10-year results from randomised trials by the Coronary Artery Bypass Graft Surgery Trialists Collaboration. *Lancet* 1994; **344**: 563–570.

12 Echt DS, Liebson PR, Mitchell LB *et al.* Mortality and morbidity in patients receiving encainide, flecainide or placebo. *N Engl J Med* 1991; **324**: 781–788.

13 Doval HC, Nul DR, Grancelli HO *et al.* Randomised trial of low dose amiodarone in severe congestive heart failure. *Lancet* 1994; **344**: 493–498.

14 Podrid PJ. Amiodarone: reevaluation of an old drug. *Ann Intern Med* 1995; **122**: 689–700.

Patients who do not Respond to Treatment

SUMMARY POINTS

- Patients with intractable heart failure can suffer from cachexia, atrophy of the body organs and changes to skeletal muscle
- Angiotensin-converting enzyme inhibitors in these patients should be used in doses shown to be effective in the large clinical trials
- A combination of diuretics, including potassium-sparing agents, helps to keep hyponatraemia and hypokalaemia in check
- Positive inotropic drugs should be used with caution, and only digoxin is available for oral treatment

A substantial proportion of patients with heart failure progress to severe disease, usually associated with enlargement of the left ventricle, worsening and persisting symptoms, raised venous pressure and peripheral oedema. Tachycardia is often present. Functional mitral regurgitation can occur as a consequence of dilatation of the mitral ring in conjunction with enlargement of the left ventricle. Mild pulmonary hypertension is often present and can lead to tricuspid regurgitation and a V wave in the jugular venous pressures. Elevated venous pressure is more often a consequence of salt and water retention in the body rather than right ventricular failure. Hepatic engorgement and oedema of the gastrointestinal tract can cause abdominal discomfort.

Intractable heart failure

Symptomatology

The symptoms of severe heart failure are fatigue, lethargy and shortness of breath. Patients who experience them are usually unable to continue their simple daily activities. The 1994 revisions to the New York Heart Association (NYHA) classification of functional capacity in patients with diseases of the heart describe class III as: 'Patients with cardiac disease resulting in marked limitation of physical activity. They are comfortable at rest. Less than ordinary activity causes fatigue, palpitation, despair, or anginal pains.'[1] Class IV is described as: 'Patients with cardiac disease resulting in the inability to carry out any physical activity without discomfort. Symptoms of heart failure or the anginal syndrome may be present. If any physical activity is undertaken, discomfort is increased.'

> Patients who experience symptoms of heart failure are usually unable to continue their simple daily activities

The new classification includes an assessment of abnormalities of the heart. Grade C is objective evidence of moderately severe cardiovascular disease, and grade D objective evidence of severe cardiovascular disease. Patients with severe, intractable or even terminal heart failure are grade 3C or above.

Pathophysiology

Severe or terminal heart failure has many features in common with other long-term chronic disabling diseases such as rheumatoid arthritis or cancer. Cachexia or atrophy of the body organs is a common feature. In particular, there are marked changes in skeletal muscle not only in the leg but throughout the body, including the diaphragm. These are not merely the consequence of repetitive ischaemia or rest atrophy, but appear to be specific and typical of the response to severe heart failure.

The principal cause of atrophy is thought to be activation of the neurohormonal and cytokine systems. Increases in insulin insensitivity, growth hormone, catecholamines, angiotensin II and cytokines such as tumour necrosis factor-α, interleukins and nitric oxide all play a role. Skeletal muscle abnormalities are the cause of the reduction in strength, and almost certainly of the tiredness and fatigue, seen in heart failure patients.

> Skeletal muscle abnormalities are the cause of the reduction in strength, and almost certainly of the tiredness and fatigue, seen in heart failure patients

In severe heart failure, blood flow to the limbs is restricted on exercise. Blood flow to the kidney may also be reduced, even at rest. Mild renal failure, demonstrated as an increase in plasma urea and creatinine, is common.

Management

Patients with intractable heart failure usually require management which involves the primary physician, hospital physician and cardiologist. In some countries, heart failure clinics have been developed to handle this difficult medical and human problem.

General support and advice from the general practitioner is needed, as it is in other forms of heart failure. Particular attention needs to be paid to body weight as a measure of salt and water retention. Severe limitation of salt intake is unpleasant and probably unacceptable, but patients should be encouraged not to add salt directly to their food or to use too much salt in cooking. Travel on aeroplanes is likely to be difficult and advice is needed. Pregnancy is dangerous to the mother, is unlikely to be successful if conception occurs, and should be vigorously discouraged.

> General support and advice from the general practitioner is needed, as it is in other forms of heart failure

Treatment

Available treatments for the patient with intractable heart failure are shown in Table 12.1. Medical therapy involves the careful use and manipulation of the many available drugs. Treatment must be tailored to the individual patient, according to symptoms, haemodynamics and pathology. In general, patients will already be receiving diuretics and angiotensin-converting enzyme (ACE) inhibitors. Many will be taking digoxin, even if they are in sinus rhythm.

The dose of ACE inhibitor should be increased to that shown to be beneficial in large clinical trials (Chapter 8) and titrated not directly against blood pressure, but more against symptoms. Low blood pressure is not an indication for altering treatment or reducing the dose of an ACE inhibitor unless hypotension is linked to symptoms. Dizziness on standing is an indication for a reduction in the dose of ACE inhibitor, or a reduction in the dose of diuretic if the patient is over diuresed.

TABLE 12.1 Severe heart failure: augmentation of standard treatment for chronic heart failure.

Intravenous drugs	Diuretics or combination of diuretics
	Nitrates
	Positive inotropes — dopamine/dobutamine
Fluid control	Haemofiltration
	Peritoneal dialysis or haemodialysis
Devices	ICD or pacing
	Intraaortic balloon pump
	Ventricular assist device
	Total artificial heart
Surgery	CABG for 'hibernation' or valve surgery
	Cardiomyoplasty
	Transplantation

The dose of ACE inhibitor should be increased to that shown to be beneficial in large clinical trials and titrated not directly against blood pressure, but against symptoms

Large doses of loop diuretics can contribute to tiredness and lethargy. If possible, the dose of frusemide should not be increased beyond 120 mg b.d. Combinations of diuretics are often useful: some patients benefit from a combination such as bendrofluazide 5 mg once daily plus amiloride 5 mg once daily and frusemide 80 mg in the morning and 80 mg in the evening.

Patients with severe heart failure often have low plasma sodium and potassium. The hypokalaemia may persist despite the use of an ACE inhibitor. In such cases, the use of a combination of diuretics (including potassium-sparing agents such as amiloride) appears to confer additional benefits. Careful attention must be paid to the plasma electrolytes, including regular measurement.

Some recent evidence suggests that adding the diuretics spironoletone and metolazone is advantageous. At first sight, the use of spironoletone may appear illogical as the patient is already taking an ACE inhibitor, which should inhibit the angiotensin pathways. However, there is some escape from this biological pathway in patients with severe heart failure, and plasma aldosterone often remains high despite the use of an ACE inhibitor.

Metolazone is a powerful diuretic which acts partly on the proximal tubule. Adding it to loop diuretics or a combination of diuretics is a useful practice of last resort in order to control sodium and water retention. However, metolazone can cause a large diuresis and should be used with caution. Patients often benefit from a small dose, such as 2.5 mg given 2 days each week or at longer periods.

Occasional patients appear to require regular doses of metolazone, but they can often be maintained on combinations of less powerful diuretics.

> Patients often benefit from a small dose of metolazone, such as 2.5 mg given 2 days each week or at longer periods

Positive inotropic drugs

Small doses of a β_2-agonist such as oral salbutamol can initiate a diuresis, as can intravenous treatment with frusemide, dopamine or a positive inotropic drug such as dobutamine. Transient use of a positive inotropic drug can be advantageous when patients are admitted to hospital with retention of sodium and water and a diuresis cannot be contrived by the use of powerful diuretics.

In general, positive inotropic drugs should be used with caution and not continued long-term. The evidence for benefit from pulsed therapy with dobutamine is controversial, but a recent report indicates some advantage.[2] Most positive inotropic drugs investigated have been shown to increase mortality. Milrinone, amrinone, vesarinone, flosequinan, ibopamine and pimbobendan have all failed to come on to the market because of a probable associated increase in mortality, particularly among patients already receiving digoxin.

> Most positive inotropic drugs investigated have been shown to increase mortality

The mechanism of harm is either the induction of an arrhythmia or progressive damage and necrosis of cardiac cells due to increased stress or mechanical load put upon contracting myocytes. For this reason, no positive inotropic drug other than digoxin is available for oral treatment. Salbutamol can be used, but is not indicated by regulatory authorities for the treatment of severe heart failure.

Haemofiltration, haemodialysis and peritoneal dialysis

In the very small number of patients in whom diuresis cannot be contrived by any combination of drugs, it is reasonable to consider interventional treatments such as haemofiltration, haemodialysis and peritoneal dialysis. These should be regarded not as a means of providing a permanent form of treatment, but rather as a way of altering the body's response and initiating a diuresis. Although there have been several reports of benefit, the numbers of patients studied have been small. Embarking on such a course requires careful discussion with the patient.

> Haemofiltration, haemodialysis and peritoneal dialysis should be regarded not as a means of providing a permanent form of treatment, but rather as a way of altering the body's response and initiating a diuresis

Cardiac surgery

By the time heart failure is considered intractable, the possible advantages of cardiac surgery should already have been considered. Occasionally, patients with recent-onset intractable heart failure benefit from surgery. Known valve disorders, such as aortic stenosis and mitral regurgitation, should certainly lead to investigations, or at least consideration of surgery. However, there appears to be no decisive advantage from surgery in patients with large ventricles, because the myocardium will have undergone extensive, usually irreversible damage.

Recently, there has been considerable interest in so-called hibernating myocardium, a condition in which the contractile function of the muscle is diminished in the presence of chronically reduced coronary flow. The hypothesis is that patients who exhibit it can benefit from coronary artery bypass surgery. Although there have been no controlled trials, several observational studies suggest its efficacy and it should be considered as an option.

Cardiomyoplasty

Cardiomyoplasty involves wrapping muscles from the back around the failing ventricle. Stimulation of the skeletal muscle in carefully selected patterns over time transforms it into slow-fibre-type skeletal muscle which can be stimulated, often on alternate beats, to aid the ejection of blood from the ventricle. No controlled trials have been reported, but observational data suggest an improvement in haemodynamics and symptoms. Patients who should be considered for this procedure are listed in Table 12.2.

TABLE 12.2 Considerations in selecting patients for cardiomyoplasty.
• Probably not if over 70 years
• Not on intravenous drugs
• Stable by NYHA class for one month
• CTR not greater than 60%
• Vital capacity not less than 60% of expected
• Mitral regurgitation less than grade 1
• Not in atrial fibrillation
• No diffuse coronary heart disease
• Pulmonary systolic pressure less than 45 mmHg
• Right ventricular ejection fraction >35%

A variant is to wrap skeletal muscle around the aorta, providing an additional pump to transmit blood around the circulation.

Ventricular assist devices

An artificial heart has been the goal of research workers for many years. The major problems in achieving it have been infection, rejection and thrombosis. Several new models of artificial heart appear to be more successful than previous attempts. They do not replace the native heart, which is not removed from the chest, but transmit blood from the failing ventricle directly to the aorta. The technique is still experimental, but interest and enthusiasm are increasing.

> New models of artificial hearts do not replace the native heart, which is not removed from the chest, but transmit blood from the failing ventricle directly to the aorta

Cardiac transplantation

Cardiac transplantation has been available since 1972 and is known to be effective. The indications and contraindications are shown in Table 12.3. The outcome is shown in Figure 12.1. Patients need to be selected carefully for this procedure as the number of hearts available in the UK is small (approximately 400 per year). It therefore follows that cardiac transplantation is not a major long-term solution to the problem of severe intractable heart failure. Furthermore, it is associated with long-term complications (Table 12.4).

TABLE 12.3 Contraindications to heart transplantation.

Age over 60. Careful consideration over 55 years
Pulmonary vascular resistance over 6–8 Wood units
Mean transpulmonary gradient >15 mmHg
Pulmonary artery systolic pressure >60 mmHg
Creatinine clearance <50 ml/min; serum creatinine >200 μmol/l
Active infection
Active ulcer disease
Severe diabetes with end-organ damage
History of drug abuse or excessive alcohol consumption
Severe psychological disturbance
Liver impairment, serum bilirubin >25 μmol/l, SGOT twice normal

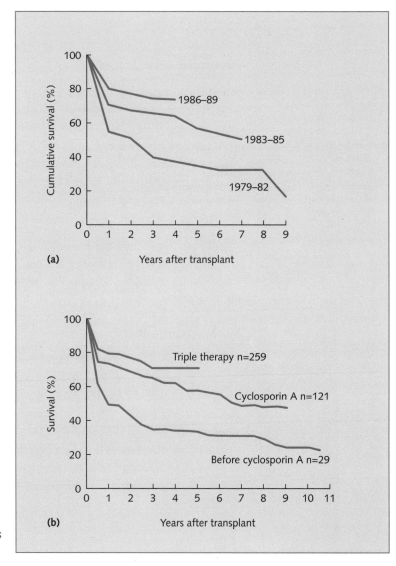

FIG. 12.1 Heart transplantation: (a) survival; (b) immunosuppression.

Cardiac transplantation is not a major long-term solution to the problem of severe intractable heart failure

Future ideas

The long-term solution to the problem of intractable heart failure probably does not lie with drugs, surgery or interventional procedures. Ideally, heart failure and the progression of ventricular damage should be prevented or delayed. If it turns out that progression is due to continuing loss of myocytes by necrosis or apoptosis, novel drugs may be used to inhibit those processes in future. Alternatively, myocardial cells might be stimulated to hypertrophy or to divide. Advances in molecular biology show that these suggestions are no longer in the realms of science fiction, but clinical application is probably at least a decade away.

Ideally, heart failure and the progression of ventricular damage should be prevented or delayed

TABLE 12.4 Long-term complications of heart transplantation.

- Infection
- Atherosclerosis 30–40% at 5 years
- Malignancy 15% at 5 years
- Renal failure 4% at 5 years
- Rejection

Reference

1 The Criteria Committee of the New York Heart Association. 1994 revisions to classification of functional capacity and objective assessment of patients with diseases of the heart. *Circulation* 1994; 90: 644–645.

Prevention of Heart Failure

SUMMARY POINTS

- Preventive strategies can be aimed either at the high-risk individual or at a whole population
- Strategies to control blood pressure and limit the progression of ischaemic heart disease offer an opportunity to prevent chronic heart failure
- There is evidence to suggest that the treatment of asymptomatic left ventricular dysfunction with angiotensin-converting enzyme inhibitors slows the progression of the disease
- Fast action after myocardial infarction is required if muscle loss is to be minimized
- Discouraging high-risk behaviour, for example smoking and a high-fat diet, may reduce the occurrence of heart failure

Rationale for prevention

Chronic heart failure (CHF) remains one of the most challenging conditions in modern medicine. Only angiotensin-converting enzyme (ACE) inhibitors have been shown conclusively to improve survival to a substantial degree, and the outlook remains poor even with optimal therapy. By the time advanced heart failure develops, mortality approaches 40% in 1 year — higher than for most forms of cancer. Because the scope for influencing the long-term outcome of heart failure is so limited, attention has turned instead to prevention.

Even with modern treatment, the prognosis for heart failure is worse than that for many forms of cancer

There are two aspects to prevention: one targetted towards the individual and one directed towards public health. An approach intended to benefit the individual patient requires screening to identify those who are at the highest risk (since it is difficult to improve the outlook in patients who are already at low risk), whereas a public health point of view calls for the introduction of preventive measures in the wider population. As the epidemiologist Geoffrey Rose pointed out in 1981, there is a 'prevention paradox': measures that bring large benefits to the community offer little to each participating individual.[1]

> Measures that bring large benefits to the community offer little to each participating individual

Programmes are already in place in many parts of the UK to screen for common, serious diseases, including breast and cervical cancer. Others have been set up to identify patients with important risk factors such as hypercholesterolaemia and hypertension. The rationale is that early identification of these conditions allows earlier treatment which, in turn, improves the prognosis in established disease and may even prevent overt disease developing at all. Intuitively, this seems a reasonable approach, and well-man and well-woman clinics have flourished in recent years.

The development of these preventive strategies has had major financial implications and places an additional burden on already over-stretched medical and ancillary services. If we wish to consider extending the net to include the prevention of heart failure, the extra workload has to be justified. Heart failure certainly has an enormous impact on resources and on patients' lives, so there is no doubt that it is sufficiently serious to merit attempts at prevention. However, we have to establish whether it is possible to identify those at risk of developing symptomatic heart failure and then intervene effectively to prevent or delay its onset.

Current knowledge about heart failure and implications for its prevention

Studies of the aetiology and natural history of heart failure raise a number of important points relevant to prevention. First, the majority of cases of clinical heart failure appear to arise as a result of coronary artery disease or hypertension, with rheumatic valve disease and dilated cardiomyopathy accounting for most of the remainder. The implication is that strategies to control blood pressure and limit the progression of ischaemic heart disease seem to offer the best chance of preventing the development of ventricular damage.

> Most cases of left ventricular (LV) dysfunction are due to ischaemic heart disease or hypertension

The second key point is that even in apparently stable chronic left ventricular (LV) dysfunction, there is a tendency for remorseless deterioration, largely independent of further insults to the myocardium. This explains the scenario of late heart failure developing years after a previous myocardial infarction (MI) and suggests that there is a recognizable latent phase during the development of heart failure, which may be amenable to intervention. The next question is whether effective forms of intervention are available.

LV dysfunction is a progressive condition. Overt heart failure may develop months or years after the initial insult

Intervention: evidence from the trials

There are clearly periods in the evolution of heart failure which provide windows of opportunity for prevention if effective strategies are available. It may be possible to intervene at the first sign of heart failure, if this can be shown to prevent or retard the subsequent decline in functional capacity. It might also be possible to identify patients with ventricular damage but minimal symptoms, and intervene before overt heart failure has had a chance to develop. Finally, and best of all, it may be possible to prevent the damage which initiates the process in the first place. In most cases, this would mean preventing myocardial infarction.

Treatment of early heart failure and asymptomatic LV dysfunction

Heart failure is a progressive condition. Mortality increases exponentially as functional class declines, and management becomes increasingly problematical. Landmark studies, such as the Cooperative North Scandinavian Enalapril Survival Study (CONSENSUS) in the 1980s,[2] established beyond doubt the value of ACE inhibitors in moderate and severe cardiac failure. The logical development was to extend this work to look at the treatment of less advanced heart failure in a similar way.

The Studies of Left Ventricular Dysfunction (SOLVD) trial was a two-part study designed to test the theory that ACE inhibitors would prove to be beneficial in patients with mild degrees of heart failure, and in those with ventricular dysfunction but no symptoms.

The first part, the SOLVD treatment arm, looked at patients with mild heart failure and reduced LV ejection fraction.[3] In the past, this group would usually have been treated solely with diuretics, partly in the mistaken belief that so-called early or mild heart failure is a benign condition, and partly through lack of evidence of an effective alternative. SOLVD demonstrated an alarming mortality (almost 40% within 4 years), and a high rate of hospitalization for CHF (18% in the same period) in the placebo group. Treatment with enalapril resulted in a 16% reduction in mortality, and a 28% reduction in the need for hospitalization because of new or worsening heart failure. Furthermore, the progressive ventricular dilatation observed in the placebo group was prevented by treatment with the ACE inhibitor.

> Mild heart failure has an alarming morbidity and mortality. ACE inhibitors should be introduced early in the course of heart failure

This study provides the rationale for the introduction of ACE inhibitors at the earliest sign of heart failure. The target dose should be equivalent to those proved effective in this and other trials (enalapril 10 mg b.d. or similar). These doses seem high to many physicians, but are usually well-tolerated and are known to reduce mortality and prevent progression to more advanced CHF.

A period of asymptomatic LV dysfunction precedes the development of asymptomatic heart failure. Again, this is a condition with an appreciable mortality and a significant risk of progression to heart failure.

In the SOLVD prevention arm, treatment with enalapril reduced the risk of the development of heart failure by 37%, and reduced the need for hospitalization because of heart failure to a similar extent.[4] The progressive ventricular dilatation seen in the placebo group was also reduced, but the study was unable to show a significant reduction in total mortality.

The important message is that ACE inhibitors slow down the rate of progression of ventricular dysfunction during the preclinical phase of heart failure, and in the longer term may have the potential significantly to affect the incidence of heart failure in the general population. Again, it is important that the doses used reflect those proven to be effective in major trials.

> ACE inhibitors reduce the progression of asymptomatic LV dysfunction

The true prevalence of minimally symptomatic LV dysfunction within the community is not yet known for certain, although it is the subject of intensive research, but the case for mass treatment of asymptomatic LV dysfunction is probably stronger than that for the treatment of mild hypertension.

> The case for screening for and treating asymptomatic LV dysfunction is stronger than that for treating mild hypertension

One of the main obstacles to the introduction of such a strategy is the difficulty of identifying patients with asymptomatic LV dysfunction, as they are by definition unlikely to present to their general practitioner. Unlike hypertension, there are no simple clinical findings which predict the need for treatment. It would therefore be necessary to screen actively for the presence of LV dysfunction in the community. Mass screening of LV function is associated with many difficulties, largely due to problems with methodology and with defining what constitutes abnormality. Techniques which measure LV function directly, such as echocardiography, are time-consuming and relatively expensive, making it doubtful they could ever be introduced outside clinical studies for routine use. The search is therefore on for alternative, more practical techniques for screening large populations. To date, serological markers such as the natriuretic peptides or widely available tools such as the standard 12-lead electrocardiogram seem to hold the most promise.

Myocardial infarction

The treatment of patients following MI has probably been studied more intensively than any other sphere of medicine, and has led to some major advances in the last couple of decades. MI is one of the most important and direct causes of heart failure, and a number of these studies are directly relevant to the question of heart failure prevention.

Thrombolysis

Despite heated debates about the advantages of alternative agents (notably streptokinase versus tissue plasminogen activator), studies have consistently shown that the key to maximizing the benefits of thrombolysis is to administer it as quickly as possible. Rapid restoration of coronary patency is the most important determinant of early myocardial function, and a patent infarct-related artery appears to protect from harmful ventricular remodelling.

It is appropriate for general practitioners in remote areas to initiate thrombolytic therapy, but in general the most important role for primary care is to ensure rapid transfer of patients to a suitable environment for them to receive thrombolysis — usually a coronary care unit. It is hard to over-emphasize the importance of avoiding unnecessary delays. Most damage is complete within 4 h of complete coronary occlusion, although the time-window may be a little longer if there is an alternative collateral supply, or if coronary occlusion is incomplete or intermittent.

> The time-delay to thrombolysis is more important than the choice of thrombolytic agent

ACE inhibitors

If thrombolysis was the success story of the 1980s in the treatment of MI, ACE inhibitors have been the most important advance so far in the 1990s. These drugs were originally evaluated for the treatment of severe heart failure, but proved so successful that attention turned to other potential indications.

The Survival and Ventricular Enlargement (SAVE) trial showed that long-term treatment with captopril improved survival (by 19%) and reduced the incidence of overt heart failure (by 22%) in patients with significant ventricular dysfunction following MI.[5] It was followed by further studies which confirmed that ACE inhibitors also offer protection to high-risk patients with clinical evidence of heart failure.[6] The survival advantage increased with greater duration of treatment, suggesting that long-term treatment with ACE inhibitors may be necessary to maximize their benefits.

The position in low-risk patients with relatively preserved LV function following MI is much less clear, as this group has never been properly evaluated in a long-term trial. CONSENSUS II showed a tendency towards increased mortality when intravenous enalapril was administered to unselected MI patients around the time of admission to hospital.[7] This result argues against the use of ACE inhibition in patients without LV dysfunction or heart failure after MI.

More recently, a number of large-scale studies have randomized unselected patients to short-term treatment with ACE inhibitors following MI, and were able to demonstrate improvements of survival in the order of a few lives for every 1000 patients treated.[8, 9] However, because it is not known whether continuing treatment in these unselected populations would have resulted in accumulating survival benefits, most physicians still reserve ACE inhibitors for larger infarcts. Doses should reflect those used in trials (for example, captopril 50 mg t.d.s., rampril 5 mg b.d.), and treatment should be continued indefinitely, if tolerated.

> ACE inhibitors are of proven benefit in patients with heart failure or LV dysfunction following MI. Treatment should be long-term, and probably indefinite, in doses that reflect those proved to be effective in clinical trials

Prevention of ischaemic events

Ischaemic heart disease accounts for the majority of cases of systolic heart failure seen in the UK, and recurrent infarction is an important factor in the progression of established LV dysfunction. It is clear then that prevention of ischaemic events, particularly MI, could have a major impact on the incidence of heart failure. The ideal strategy would prevent the development of coronary atheroma — overwhelmingly the main cause of infarction.

One of the first studies to address this issue was the Multiple Risk Factor Intervention Trial (MRFIT), which compared intensive stepped care, including treatment for hypertension, with routine care in the community.[10] It was unable to show a significant reduction in coronary terms in the special intervention group over a 7-year follow-up; however, it was suggested that potential benefits may have been masked by the unexpectedly large improvement in risk behaviour during the study in the normal care group.

More recently, evidence has emerged that long-term treatment with ACE inhibitors may reduce ischaemic events in survivors of MI, and in patients with reduced ejection fraction.[11, 12] This has not been a universal finding in ACE inhibitor trials but, interestingly, has been observed in the two investigations with the longest duration of treatment (SAVE and SOLVD). This could be interpreted as indicating that ACE inhibitors have a slow-acting effect, perhaps on the coronary vasculature or through inhibition of the renin–angiotensin system. While the true significance of the finding is unclear, it provides a further stimulus for the early use of

ACE inhibitors in appropriate groups, and may explain some of their beneficial effects.

> Evidence has emerged that long-term treatment with ACE inhibitors may reduce ischaemic events in survivors of MI, and in patients with reduced ejection fraction

Finally, a great deal of attention has concentrated on the treatment of hyperlipidaemia, a further major risk factor for coronary disease. Early trials of lipid-lowering agents (mainly fibrates) in the primary prevention of ischaemic heart disease achieved a certain notoriety.[13, 14] There was evidence of a reduction in cardiovascular events, but unfortunately this was at the expense of increased all-cause mortality, with a particular excess of violent deaths. This issue sparked enormous controversy, but was too consistent a finding to be dismissed simply as chance. In the UK, it effectively removed lipid-lowering from the agenda of most physicians for primary prevention, with the unfortunate knock-on effect that it also reduced interest in lipid-lowering in other, more appropriate groups.

All this changed in 1994 with the publication of the Scandinavian 4S Study.[15] For the first time it was shown that drug treatment could substantially reduce total mortality and cardiovascular events in patients with mild and moderate hyperlipidaemia (cholesterol 5.5–7.5 mmol/l). The benefit was additional to the effects of diet (all patients followed a lipid-lowering diet for 6 months before treatment was initiated).

There were two key differences between 4S and the previous studies. First, 4S looked at the secondary prevention of major ischaemic events in a relatively high-risk cohort with established coronary disease; second, the drug used was one of the statins, which reduce cholesterol levels more effectively than previous agents. Although heart failure was not a specified end-point, it is likely that reduction of ischaemic events would translate into a lower risk of ventricular damage and ultimately heart failure.

The message is that all patients with a history of ischaemic heart disease, and particularly MI, should have their serum cholesterol concentration measured. Those with a level greater than 5.5 mmol/l should be advised to follow a lipid-lowering diet and if levels remain high, a statin should be prescribed to reduce the level to below 5.0 mmol/l.

> Lipid-lowering therapy with a statin reduces clinical events in patients with established coronary disease and raised cholesterol levels

Interestingly, the magnitude of benefit with treatment in the 4S study was similar in all subjects, regardless of the cholesterol level. It has now been shown that survivors of myocardial infarction benefit from cholesterol reduction, even if their baseline values are within the normal range.[16] This may be particularly relevant in high-risk patients with multivessel coronary disease, or previous bypass-grafting. It is debatable whether it is necessary or desirable for patients to follow a diet for a period of time before receiving drug therapy. The evidence that dietary measures reduce cardiac events is much weaker and may waste potential therapeutic time. Furthermore it is unlikely that dieting alone normalizes cholesterol levels in excess of 7.0 mmol/l. In appropriate patients, it seems reasonable to initiate drug treatment immediately.

Latterly, the West of Scotland Coronary Prevention Study (WOSCOPS) has widened the scope of lipid-lowering treatment by showing benefits in patients without coronary disease. However, statins are expensive drugs and the cost effectiveness of this approach is uncertain. For the present lipid-lowering drugs should be reserved for higher risk patients in the context of primary prevention.[17]

> In appropriate patients, it seems reasonable to initiate drug treatment immediately

Hypertension

The Framingham study raised the possibility that heart failure might be largely preventable through early and aggressive treatment of hypertension.[18] It was already accepted that the treatment of the relatively few patients with malignant hypertension was overwhelmingly beneficial, but it was equally obvious that this would have little impact on the incidence of heart failure in the population overall. Interest focused instead on the much greater number of patients with moderate and, particularly, mild hypertension who make up the majority of the at-risk population. The definitions of mild and moderate hypertension are rather arbitrary, but diastolic pressures consistently below 110–115 mmHg would generally be classed as mild, and pressures of 115–130 mmHg as moderate.

Many studies conducted over the last 30 years have convincingly demonstrated that reducing hypertension can lead to a decrease in the incidence of cerebrovascular disease by as much as a third. Unfortunately, however, such treatment has no significant impact on the incidence of either MI or total mortality.

> Unfortunately, drug treatment has no impact on the incidence of MI or on total mortality in patients with mild hypertension

There are a number of possible explanations for this rather disappointing finding. First, as the risk of cardiovascular disease (MI or CHF) developing in any given individual during the course of the studies was relatively low, it was difficult to show a statistically significant reduction in absolute risk. In this situation, minor adverse effects of the study drugs can quickly begin to outweigh the benefits, and both thiazides and β-blockers have metabolic effects which might theoretically predispose to acceleration of atherosclerosis. A further possibility is that reductions in ischaemic heart disease mortality in certain subgroups may have been marked by unfavourable effects in others, and that more selective treatment may still be beneficial.

It is also clear that hypertension is a chronic disease, and very prolonged antihypertensive treatment may be necessary before the full benefits emerge. A study looking at a minimum of 10 years of therapy in large numbers of patients may be needed to show this, but is unlikely to be carried out.

A number of newer antihypertensive agents have potential advantages in their mechanisms of action, or side-effect profiles, compared with older drugs, and might improve the outlook even in mild hypertension. ACE inhibitors, for example, have been shown to cause regression of vascular and myocardial hypertrophy, and also to modulate the activity of the renin–angiotensin system. α-Blockers have a beneficial effect on the lipid profile. Although each of these (more expensive) agents has its enthusiasts, there is no evidence as yet that they result in a reduction in actual clinical events in patients with hypertension.

> ACE inhibitors have been shown to cause regression of vascular and myocardial hypertrophy, and also to modulate the activity of the renin–angiotensin system

The situation with regard to calcium channel blockers provides a particularly interesting example of the difficulties associated with determining the effects of long-term treatment. These drugs are widely used in hypertension (and angina), not least because of their good safety profile. Recently, however, there has been a report associating short-acting calcium channel blockers with increased risk of MI.[19] The jury is still out on this issue, but it is a salutary reminder that even well-established forms of treatment can have unsuspected side-effects.

For the moment, it is difficult to recommend treating mild hypertension using any agent with the sole aim of preventing heart failure. Most physicians will continue to institute treatment for the prevention of stroke, despite the small reduction in individual risk, in the knowledge that this policy could substantially reduce the incidence of stroke in the population. However, to avoid overtreatment it is worth noting the recommendations of the British Hypertension Society working party that treatment should be initiated only in patients whose diastolic blood pressure averages 100 mmHg or more over 3–4 months.[20] In the first instance, therapy should be with a β-blocker or a diuretic; other agents are only to be added if these are contra-indicated or poorly tolerated.

Putting it into practice

The question arises of how to translate the results of clinical trials into a practical strategy for preventing heart failure. Selecting extremely high-risk individuals appears to be an appropriate and efficient use of medical resources, but the impact on the burden of heart failure is inevitably small.

The alternative approach is mass action, which offers relatively little to the individuals involved (because most of them are at low risk anyway), but has a significant effect on population health. The simplest strategy is to encourage the public to avoid potentially harmful factors, such as saturated fat, tobacco and sloth. The advantage of this approach is that it is both cheap and safe. However, in practice, it is difficult to change the behaviour of society through advice alone; there must be an additional incentive for change, which may be social (such as the current fashion for fitness), economic (such as increasing tax on tobacco) or legislative (such as banning tobacco advertising).

> In practice, it is difficult to change the behaviour of society through advice alone; there must be an additional incentive for change

An alternative form of mass action is to add a new, beneficial factor (such as long-term medication) to large numbers of relatively low-risk individuals. In contrast to the avoidance strategy, this is expensive; more importantly, such interventions may carry small risks which can easily outweigh their potential advantages. The increased overall mortality seen with clofibrate therapy in the World Health Organization trial of lipid-lowering in primary prevention (in the face of a 26% reduction in non-fatal MI) is a vivid example of this phenomenon.[21]

The mega-trials have introduced a third strategy, which involves screening for and treating patients with an intermediate level of risk. The SOLVD study provides a paradigm of this approach, as the benefits of ACE inhibitor therapy to individual patients were small (particularly in the prevention arm), but the potential benefits to the population were relatively large.

Role of primary care

So, what is the role for primary care in the prevention of heart failure where traditionally there has been a responsibility to the individual patient above all else, but where increasingly this has to be balanced with the need to achieve set targets for public health dictated by the government? The following approach is suggested as a starting point. An initial assessment is made of the patient's baseline risk of developing heart failure, the results of which dictate the strategy for prevention.

Assessment of risk

The risk of an individual developing heart failure depends on the probability of established (silent) LV dysfunction, and the likelihood of cardiovascular events (ventricular damage) occurring in the short term. In practice, this usually means looking at risk factors for ischaemic heart disease. The approach to prevention differs according to the findings.

Major risk factors for ischaemic heart disease are:
1   smoking;
2   family history of premature ischaemic heart disease;
3   hypertension;
4   diabetes;
5   hypercholesterolaemia.

Tailored preventive strategies

Low-risk patients

> *Characteristics of low-risk patients*
> Low probability of established LV dysfunction
> Low risk of cardiovascular events within 5 years
>   No known ischaemic heart disease
>   0 or 1 risk factors

Strictly speaking, many low-risk individuals are not patients at all, as they have no manifest illness. They have the least to gain from prevention, and the most to lose if attempts at prevention have unforeseen side-effects. It is particularly important that any intervention intended to protect this population must be entirely safe.

The general practitioner has two important roles in such cases — promotion of a healthy lifestyle and risk factor surveillance.

With regard to promoting a healthy lifestyle, it is not possible to separate the prevention of heart failure from the prevention of cardiovascular disease in general, as heart failure may develop as a consequence of hypertensive or ischaemic damage. Most current advice about healthy lifestyles is tailored to the avoidance of cardiovascular disease, because this is the biggest killer from early middle age onwards. Smoking is the most potent and readily correctable risk factor, and has to be forcefully discouraged. It is extremely difficult to change long-established patterns of behaviour, but general practitioners are in a uniquely powerful position to influence the attitudes of their patients towards this and other risk factors.

Although there is little objective evidence that diet, exercise and weight make any significant difference to the risk of coronary disease in an individual patient, at least in the short term, general advice should be given.

> General practitioners are in a uniquely powerful position to influence the attitudes of their patients towards smoking and other risk factors

With regard to risk factor surveillance, the major modifiable risk factors for ischaemic heart disease other than smoking are hypertension and hyperlipidaemia. Most — if not all — primary care practices should already have a policy which ensures that all their patients have their blood pressure measured at least once every 2–3 years. This can usually coincide with attendance at the practice for other reasons. Despite the striking epidemiological importance of hypertension, treatment of mild blood pressure has a disappointing impact on the incidence of MI, and therefore also on the incidence of heart failure. This is not the case in more severe hypertension, however, and this alone provides the incentive to continue screening.

A strong association has also been established between dyslipidaemias and coronary events within the population, and many general practitioners already measure cholesterol levels routinely in all their adult patients. A low-fat diet should be recommended in the presence of hyperlipidaemia, but there is little evidence to support instituting lipid-lowering drug therapy in an otherwise low-risk group.

It is important that general practitioners are seen to show an interest in avoidable risk factors (despite uncertainty about the absolute value of some of these measures) because otherwise patients can hardly be expected to have much enthusiasm. Once patients focus their attention towards their risk factors, it becomes more likely that they will modify their behaviour. The decline in cardiovascular mortality seen in the USA and Australasia proves that changes are possible, although their mechanism and time-course are unclear.

> *Management of low-risk patients*
> Promotion of a healthy lifestyle
> Risk factor surveillance

Intermediate-risk patients

> *Characteristics of intermediate-risk patients*
> Low probability of established LV dysfunction
> High risk of cardiovascular events within 5 years
>   Angina pectoris (particularly unstable angina)
>   Previous MI with documentation of preserved LV function
>   Multiple risk factors (two or more)

Individuals who have an increased risk of developing heart failure are, by implication, usually also at risk of MI. The most obvious group includes patients with angina pectoris, but those with multiple cardiovascular risk factors are also included.

General advice on lifestyle (particularly smoking) is even more important in this population and should be given at every

185

opportunity. However, a number of specific measures should also be considered. Most importantly, patients known to have ischaemic heart disease should be assessed for total serum cholesterol (not necessarily fasting). Those with a level above 5.5 mmol/l should be started on a lipid-lowering diet and specific lipid-lowering therapy in the form of a statin. Lipid-lowering is proven to reduce the risk of fatal and non-fatal MI, and there is evidence that it also slows the progression (and may even induce regression) of coronary atheroma. It is now clear that the same approach can usefully be applied to the other increased risk groups even in the absence of known coronary disease.

Patients with persistent hypertension and those with long-standing diabetes should have a 12-lead electrocardiogram recorded (Chapter 6). In hypertensives, the electrocardiogram provides a crude screening tool for the identification of LV hypertrophy and, if a so-called strain pattern is found, also provides important prognostic information. Diabetics on the other hand may suffer silent infarction which can be demonstrated by the presence of pathological Q waves and characteristic ST segment changes. The presence of these features should prompt referral for further assessment by a cardiovascular physician, as these patients may already have important ventricular dysfunction. Conversely, a normal 12-lead electrocardiogram makes the presence of significant LV dysfunction unlikely.

Management of intermediate-risk patients
General measures as for low-risk patients
Investigations
   12-lead electrocardiogram
   Cholesterol
Specific measures
   Statins for hypercholesterolaemia

High-risk patients

Characteristics of high-risk patients
High probability of established LV dysfunction
High risk of cardiovascular events within 5 years
  Previous MI with documented LV dysfunction or evidence of
    heart failure
  Previous MI (particularly anterior Q-wave MI or left bundle
    branch block): no assessment of LV function made
  Previous coronary artery bypass surgery
  CHF symptoms: uncertain cause

Patients at the highest risk of developing heart failure are those with established but clinically silent LV dysfunction. Unfortunately, this population is very difficult to identify without the use of expensive and time-consuming imaging techniques such as echocardiography. Systematic screening of the population for asymptomatic ventricular dysfunction would be extremely expensive, and difficult to justify when the benefits of ACE inhibitor treatment are relatively modest.

It may be possible to narrow the field down, however, and concentrate on individuals who have had a previous MI. This group has a high prevalence of ventricular dysfunction, particularly those patients who have had an anterior Q-wave MI or who have had an infarct complicated by heart failure. It may therefore be reasonable to start an ACE inhibitor without formal assessment of LV function in such instances. In most other cases, an echocardiogram will be required in order to estimate ventricular function prior to initiating what may be lifelong therapy. Increasing provision by hospitals of open-access echo services makes this policy more practical.

Most patients should now be started on ACE inhibitor therapy prior to discharge after acute MI if there has been evidence of heart failure, or if there is objective evidence of LV dysfunction. However, there is still a large population of patients who sustained their infarct before the era of ACE inhibitors, who have unsuspected or silent ventricular dysfunction, and who are heading down the slippery slope towards overt heart failure. Treatment of this group with ACE inhibitors is known to delay the development of heart failure, and may reduce mortality.

Management of high-risk patients
General measures as for low-risk patients
Investigations as for intermediate-risk patients plus
    echocardiography for suspected LV dysfunction

Suspected or early heart failure

Physicians routinely treat mild hypertension with drugs of uncertain value (and uncertain safety). They are also happy to institute diuretic therapy in early heart failure despite a plethora of side-effects, and concerns that it may cause harmful stimulation of the renin–angiotensin system. In contrast, there is still some reluctance to institute ACE inhibitor treatment in mild cases of CHF, and to use doses lower than those known to be effective and well-tolerated. This is despite clear evidence that ACE inhibition improves mortality in patients with all classes of symptomatic heart failure, and reduces the rate of progression of symptomatic and asymptomatic LV dysfunction.

There is still some reluctance to institute ACE inhibitor treatment in mild cases of CHF, and to use doses lower than those known to be effective and well-tolerated

As we move into an era of evidence-based medicine, we should be maximizing the use of strategies known to be effective. The value of ACE inhibitors in the management of ventricular dysfunction is beyond doubt. The key to realizing their benefits is to consider using them as soon as heart failure is suspected, so that progression to more severe failure can be delayed. The clinical diagnosis of heart failure is sometimes difficult, however, and it may be preferable to obtain an objective assessment of LV function, usually by echocardiography. The advent of open-access services has made this approach more practical, and should facilitate the appropriate use of ACE inhibitors in the future.

Conclusions

The management of established heart failure remains a problem, despite advances in drug therapy in the last few years. Even with modern treatment, heart failure reduces both length and quality of life to a greater degree than almost any other chronic medical condition. This has provided the impetus to look at the prospects for prevention.

Thanks to recent studies, we know that heart failure is the end-stage of a process characterized by progressive deterioration in ventricular function. In most cases the aetiology is ischaemic heart disease or hypertension, although valvular disease and cardiomyopathy are also relevant. There is firm evidence that this cycle can be interrupted, and the onset of heart failure either delayed or prevented.

The first step in developing a preventive strategy is to assess the patient's risk, and modify the approach accordingly. All primary care practices should have a policy on risk factor surveillance and general health promotion (particularly regarding smoking) for their adult patients. Specific investigation and treatment are of value for patients judged to be at high risk of developing heart failure. Lipid-lowering drugs reduce cardiac events (and therefore prevent ventricular damage) in patients with coronary artery disease and hypercholesterolaemia. ACE inhibitors are the cornerstone of therapy in patients with significant, but silent, LV dysfunction, and in those with so-called early or mild heart failure.

> ACE inhibitors are the cornerstone of therapy in patients with significant, but silent, LV dysfunction, and in those with so-called early or mild heart failure

ACE inhibitor treatment has to be long term to maximise its benefits. Furthermore, even when treating patients with few symptoms, the doses used should reflect those proved to be effective in the major trials (Table 13.1).

TABLE 13.1 Target doses of angiotensin-converting enzyme (ACE) inhibitors used in major trials.

Drug	Total daily dose (if tolerated)	Dose frequency
Captopril	100–150 mg	b.d. or t.d.s.
Enalapril	20 mg	b.d.
Lisinopril	10 mg	o.d.
Ramipril	10 mg	b.d.
Trandolapril	1–4 mg	o.d.

It is hoped that this practical strategy is sufficiently simple to be useful to busy general practitioners. Its widespread introduction would result in a reduction in the social and economic burden of heart failure in the UK, and substantially reduce the need for hospitalization.

References

1 Rose G. Strategy of prevention: lessons from cardiovascular disease. *Br Med J* 1981; **282**: 1847–1851.

2 CONSENSUS Trial Study Group. Effects of enalapril on mortality in severe congestive heart failure. Results of the cooperative north Scandinavian enalapril survival study. *N Engl J Med* 1987; **316**: 1429–1435.

3 The SOLVD Investigators. Effect of enalapril on survival in patients with reduced left ventricular ejection fractions and congestive heart failure. *N Engl J Med* 1991; **325**: 293–302.

4 The SOLVD Investigators. Effect of enalapril on mortality and the development of heart failure in asymptomatic patients with reduced left ventricular ejection fractions. [Published erratum appears in *N Engl J Med* 1992; **327**: 1768] *N Engl J Med* 1992; **327**: 686–691.

5 Pfeffer MA, Braunwald E, Moye LA *et al.* Effect of captopril on mortality and morbidity in patients with left ventricular dysfunction after myocardial infarction. Results of the survival and ventricular enlargement trial. The SAVE Investigators. *N Engl J Med* 1992; **327**: 669–677.

6 The AIRE Study Investigators. Effect of ramipril on mortality and morbidity of survivors of acute myocardial infarction with clinical evidence of heart failure. *Lancet* 1993; **342**: 821–828.

7 Swedberg K, Held P, Kjekshus J, Rasmussen K, Ryden L, Wedel H. Effects of the early administration of enalapril on mortality in patients with acute myocardial infarction results of the cooperative new Scandinavian enalapril survival study 11 (CONSENSUS II). *N Engl J Med* 1992; **327**: 678–684.

8 Gruppo Italiano per lo Studio della Sopravvivenza nell'Infarto Miocardico. GISS1-3: Effects of lisinopril and transdermal glyceryl trinitrate singly and together on 6-week mortality and ventricular function after acute myocardial infarction. *Lancet* 1994; **343**: 1115–1122.

9 ISIS-4 (Fourth International Study of Infarct Survival) Collaborative Group OU. Protocol for a large simple study of the effects of oral mononitrate, of oral captopril, and of intravenous magnesium. *Am J Cardiol* 1991; **68**: 87D–100D.

10 Multiple Risk Factor Intervention Trial Research Group. Multiple risk factor intervention trial: risk factor changes and mortality results. *JAMA* 1982; **248**: 1465–1477.

11 Rutherford JD, Pfeffer MA, Moye LA *et al.* Effects of captopril on ischaemic events after myocardial infarction. *Circulation* 1994; **90**: 1731–1738.

12 Yusuf S, Pepine CJ, Garces C *et al.* Effect of enalapril on myocardial infarction and unstable angina in patients with low ejection fractions. *Lancet* 1992; **340**: 1173–1178.

13 Committee of Principal Investigators. A cooperative trial in the primary prevention of ischaemic heart disease using clofibrate. *Br Heart J* 1978; **40**: 1069–1118.

14 Frick MH, Elo O, Happa K *et al.* Helsinki heart study: primary prevention with gemfibrozil in middle-aged men with dyslipemia. *N Engl J Med* 1987; **317**: 1237–1245.

15 Scandinavian Simvastatin Survival Study Group. Randomised trial of cholesterol lowering in 4444 patients with coronary heart disease: the Scandinavian simvastatin survival study (4S). *Lancet* 1994; **344**: 1383–1389.

16 Franks MS, Pfeffer MA, Moye LA *et al.* The effect of Pravastatin on coronary events after myocardial infarction in patients with average cholesterol levels. *N Engl J Med* 1996; **335**: 1001–1009.

17 Shepherd J, Cobbe SM, Ford I *et al.* Prevention of coronary heart disease with pravastatin in men with hypercholesterolaemia. *N Engl J Med* 1995; **333**: 1301–1307.

18 Kannel WB, Castelli WP, McNamara PM, McKee PA, Feinleib M. Role of blood pressure in the development of congestive heart failure. The Framingham study. *N Engl J Med* 1972; **287:** 781–787.

19 Psaty BM, Heckbert SR, Koepsell TD *et al.* The risk of myocardial infarction associated with antihypertensive drug therapies. *JAMA* 1995; **274:** 620–625.

20 British Hypertension Society Working Party. Treating mild hypertension: agreement from the large trials. *Br Med J* 1989; **298:** 694–698.

21 Report from the Committee of Principal Investigators. A co-operative trial in the primary prevention of ischaemic heart disease using clofibrate. *Br Heart J* 1978; **40:** 1069–1118.

Index